I'm So
effing
Tired

I'm So effing Tired

Dr Amy Shah

PIATKUS

PIATKUS

First published in the United States in 2021 by Houghton Mifflin Harcourt
First published in Great Britain in 2021 by Piatkus

A CIP catalogue record for this book is available from the British Library.

ISBN: 978-0-34942-790-4

Printed and bound in Great Britain by Clays Ltd, Elcograf S.p.A.
Book design by Chrissy Kurpeski. Typeset in Arno Pro.

Papers used by Piatkus are from well-managed forests and other responsible sources.

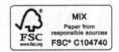

Infographics for 'Hormonal Highway' (page 25) and 'New Food Pyramid' (page 176) by
Chrissy Kurpeski, adapted from Lina Issa. Infographics for 'Optimize Your Circadian
Rhythm' (page 142) and 'Optimizing Exercise and Fasting for a Woman' (page 193)
by Chrissy Kurpeski, adapted from Ginalyn McNamara.

Piatkus
An imprint of
Little, Brown Book Group
Carmelite House
50 Victoria Embankment
London EC4Y 0DZ

An Hachette UK Company
www.hachette.co.uk

www.littlebrown.co.uk.

Contents

Introduction

Why Was I So Effing Tired?

M Y HEAD WAS SPINNING. Feeling guilty for leaving my "impromptu" 5 p.m. meeting early and equally guilt-ridden for being late to pick up my kids, I felt my heart pounding as I raced down Sixty-Seventh Avenue in Glendale, Arizona. My thoughts toggled back and forth, thinking about my hasty departure from the office, the imagined annoyance of my co-workers, and envisioning my kids waiting for me at the karate studio. I imagined the cranky front desk attendant at the studio chastising me for my tardiness and judging me for my poor mothering skills.

I was so preoccupied with my self-doubt, I didn't see the other car at the intersection until it was too late. Time stopped as the sound of metal hitting metal filled the air. My car spun out of control, three times to be exact, before colliding with the concrete divider. Another overwhelming sound of crushing metal. Every airbag in the car released at once. As soon as I came to, I could see that my arms were bloody from the shattered glass of the windshield. I was okay, but I knew the accident was my fault. And it was the perfect metaphor for my life at the time. I felt like I was out of control. Scratch that, *I knew* I was.

At the time of my accident — ten years ago now — I had been practically running on empty, raising two kids and studying for my medical boards while trying to build a thriving practice as an immunologist. I was overtired, overworked, and overextended. (Sound familiar?) It wasn't just about time management. It was deeper than that: my body was telling me that something was wrong with *me*. I was gaining weight inexplicably. I was cranky all the time. My energy was nonexistent. I couldn't figure out what was wrong and felt too tired to find out. And it didn't help that everyone around me told me what I was feeling was just the fact of being a busy working mom. (Ugh, can you relate?) Perhaps by divine intervention, the car accident was the wake-up call I needed to make big changes in my life.

❧

Before the accident, I felt alone in my inability to manage all of my personal and professional demands. I assumed my fatigue was just a normal and inevitable part of life. But I now know that I was wrong. And, unfortunately, I know I was not the only one who felt this way — far too many women suffer from an energy crisis, just as I did. I have had patients who worried about burning the candle at both ends and felt frazzled, overstressed, and exhausted because of it — too many to count. Maybe it's why you picked up this book. It's far too common for us to feel overstretched and overwhelmed — how can we not in this day and age? We have busy lives, juggling work with family life, all the while sidestepping nonstop distractions every day. But we aren't superhuman, and there are points in which we put too much stress on our bodies that can cause it to buckle; the body can't seem to juggle any more, and it stops working as it should.

Take my 34-year-old patient Katie, who had a busy copywriting business and two young children. Even though she worked from home, she was more stressed than ever and came to me because she was having major sleep issues that were interfering with both her work and her home life. She was so tired that she was losing focus on work, and it was worrying her since her family was dependent on her paycheck. She also was experiencing similar symptoms that I had:

- Fatigue
- Sleep disruption
- Cravings for both sweet and salty foods
- Excessive need for stimulants such as caffeine
- Vague but persistent digestive problems

Katie's story is sadly common these days. My story is, too.

Maybe you see yourself in our stories. And maybe, like us, you've been told by friends, family, and possibly even doctors that there's nothing to be done about it (except, perhaps, quitting your job or going on an extended vacation from your life — not exactly a feasible solution!). If so, you're not alone — and this book is designed with just you in mind. I am offering you a solution that can help you regain your lost energy and reclaim your life. I've developed this plan to transform my own life, and it's helped thousands of my patients. I know it can do the same for you. (In fact, you'll read more of my patients' stories here in this book.)

A BIT ABOUT ME

I'm a double-board-certified doctor of medicine who studied at Cornell, Albert Einstein, Harvard, and Columbia. But, perhaps more important, I'm a mom of two who also faced a dark place where I felt all kinds of tired. Following my accident, I worked tirelessly in creating a program that works with the woman's body to tamp down stress and boost energy. And once I created a plan that worked — and experienced a massive change in my own health — I knew I needed to share it with my patients. A part of my practice is now dedicated to helping women overcome exhaustion, and I've seen this plan work for thousands of patients. It changed my life. I believe it can change yours, too.

I never expected for this to be my life's mission. Before my energy crisis — long before I became a doctor, or a mother, or a women's health advocate — I had always been energetic. In fact, I was a ball of energy growing up in the sleepy town of Nashik, in Western India, about three hours east of Mumbai. We didn't have a car or a TV, but we lived in a town that took care of its own, and everyone in my apartment building knew and treated each other like one big, loud, hands-in-the-air dramatic but happy family.

When I was five, my parents got the opportunity to come to America, eventually settling in a sleepy, leafy suburb in Westchester, New York. The move was hard for me. Not only was there culture shock and a big learning curve as I tried to pick up the English language, but I didn't feel like I belonged. Whether it was my hand-me-down wardrobe that didn't win over my fashion-forward classmates or the fact that I walked to school instead of getting a ride like every other kid, I felt alone. Suddenly, I was the only brown person in my entire class, and to say I did not fit in was an understatement. I was teased about my clothes and my heritage. It didn't help that I was a vegetarian, either — back in the '80s, that was like having two heads. I will never forget the day when my veggie lunch was mysteriously replaced with a hamburger. (A cruel prank.)

In high school, the challenges became more serious: my loved ones were getting sick. My grandmother was dealing with diabetes and all the complications that come with it; my grandfather had it, too, and passed away young at the age of 60. My dad and all four of his brothers had been diagnosed with type 2 diabetes by the time they were in their early thirties. *How could that be,* I remember thinking, *they all seemed so healthy and fit.* Once, at a family dinner, my uncle the cardiologist warned us, as he passed the roti, "Diabetes runs rampant in families, and unfortunately our family's one of them. You all are going to get it. If we leave you nothing else — this is our gift." He laughed. He added, as if to underscore the severity of the illness, "Nobody in our family really has lived past sixty." This comment has always stuck with me — and it was perhaps the moment when I first started to wonder if our genes really were our destiny, or if we perhaps had more control over our health than we realized.

I set about learning as much as I could about the disease. I would take my grandmother to the doctor and be her translator, taking the opportunity to ask a lot of questions. I was especially interested in what role genetics versus diet and lifestyle played in our health. As I learned about diabetes and how food could be a major factor in fending off its most serious symptoms, I enlisted my dad as a guinea pig to test out some of the recommended diets. Together, we went on a series of crazy diets — high fat, low carb, vegan, paleo, Ayurvedic — to name just a few. It wasn't easy: for him, and many people like him, it is really hard to break lifelong habits. It was difficult for him to give up foods he grew up on as well as his go-to favorite comfort foods, especially his morning khakhra (wheat wafers), but he humored me and stuck with it. Eventually we found a diet plan that worked. In two years, he went from using 50 units of insulin to less than 20, and he lost about 30 pounds! This diet formed the foundation of the plan you hold in your hands today. (And don't worry, you may think you can never have the foods you love, but you can, sometimes. You'll see soon.)

This got me thinking that there was a lot of interplay between the human body, food, genetics, and lifestyle changes. I was also intrigued by metabolism: How could some people eat what they wanted and remain thin while others couldn't lose weight no matter how little they ate? (Life is not fair, right?) Inspired by my experience with my father's diet and eager to answer these questions, I applied to Cornell University's Division of Nutritional Sciences, arguably the best program of its kind. In the summers, I did research at Harvard Medical School and learned how the immune system works and how it's affected by pollutants in the modern environment. (Harvard's Boston location offered more than just an education for me: this is where my love for the Boston Red Sox and the Patriots started — and this was even before the Patriots' Tom Brady success.)

To deepen my understanding of food and the human body, I attended Albert Einstein College of Medicine, in New York City, where I met my future husband, a young, ambitious Californian who was the kindest person I have ever met (still is).

During medical school, my passion for disease prevention continued. I took a full year to devote my time principally to research in heart disease, which helped sharpen my skills in critically analyzing studies for the rest of my career. Following medical school, I chose Harvard Medical School's Beth Israel Deaconess Medical Center in Boston for my residency. I was a little burned out from medical school, and having just gotten married, my start there was brutal. The hours were worse than med school, and I found it incredibly difficult to get through the long workdays. It didn't help that Boston got dark so early so many months out of the year. I would go into work before 6 a.m. and it would be pitch-black, and then I would get out of work in the evening and, guess what, it'd be pitch-black. *Get me out of here!* I thought. I learned the hard way how our circadian rhythm could alter our mood and energy during Boston's dark winters. When people talk about seasonal affective disorder, I know what they mean. I remember feeling no excitement or passion through those Boston winters and then, just like a light switch, I would get a surge of energy when spring arrived.

Luckily, I was accepted into the Columbia immunology program two years later and we moved to New York. I was pregnant with my second child and studying immunology again. (Believe me, I see the humor in being pregnant and on that hormonal roller coaster while studying women's hormones and the immune system!) This was a formative experience for me. Both my clinical work in allergy and my science work in immunology set the stage for the book you're reading.

After many years of school and training, I was double board certified in both internal medicine and allergy/immunology. I started my practice, thrilled to put this education to use. But I quickly sensed that my special training and expertise were feeling almost wasted on the Western model of medicine and its revolving door of patients. Don't get me wrong, I *loved* interacting with patients, but I wanted to do more than just treat their problems — I wanted to help to PREVENT them, but there was not enough time. I felt burned out but also trapped as I juggled my medical practice with motherhood. We had two sweet children by this time, and my husband had his own stresses with his medical practice. I was only 32, but I was running myself ragged.

Then I had the car accident. I knew something was wrong with me. But what, exactly? Why was I so effing tired all the time?

FINDING AN ANSWER TO
THE ENERGY CRISIS

These vague but undeniable symptoms were obvious to me, but their cause was elusive to all my doctors. I kept asking my friends — the brightest colleagues from my training at Harvard and Columbia — to help me figure out why I was feeling this way. They looked at me blankly and told me I was "fine." They assured me that fatigue was "normal" for a new mother and for someone starting a new practice and said, "It's not uncommon." Worst of all, they told me that "aging" could be to blame and that my hormones may not be as "active" as they used to be. *What?! At 32?* It was the feeling of dread when I read a women's magazine and they refer to anyone over 25 as "older."

I refused to believe it. I also knew I was hardly alone in feeling this way. So many of my patients, friends, and colleagues complained of the same nagging fatigue, fogginess, and moodiness. And their sleep was . . . well, what sleep? But their symptoms have been long marginalized by their doctors. Just like me, their unexplained symptoms were dismissed and attributed to being a "new mom" or "overworked" or as a by-product of "aging." I felt like a broken record, constantly telling people about how tired I was — I was just *tired* of complaining about it. (Aren't you?)

The more I dug into the issue of fatigue in women, the more I became convinced that we have a major energy crisis on our hands. In a recent study, 15 percent of women reported that they often felt very tired or exhausted, compared to 10 percent of men.[1] And women between the ages of 18 and 44 were almost *twice as likely as men* to often feel very tired or exhausted (15.7 versus 8.7 percent).[2] What's worse, throughout medical history women (and their medical issues) have been neglected by research. (Believe it or not, the NIH didn't mandate that women be included in research studies until 1994! In other words, women have suffered from an energy crisis and hormone imbalances in general for ages with no help—their complaints always dismissed as symptoms of "getting older.") But there was nothing in the literature to support that evaluation and no definitive treatment. There is still too little scientific literature addressing this issue. I could go on about the injustices here, but that is for another book entirely . . . My point is that I was physically tired, and I was also tired that women were getting short shrift by conventional medicine and research.

By the way, as frustrating as it is that women have been marginalized by the health care system, what's worse is that minority groups are overlooked even more, and it's not necessarily about income disparity. In a 2017 study, Tina Sacks, an assistant professor of social welfare at UC Berkeley, conducted dozens of in-depth interviews and concluded that "infant mortality rates for black women with a college degree are higher than those for white women with just a high school education."[3] Black women's symptoms are often discounted by their doctors, even for celebrity patients like Serena Williams, who couldn't get a medical professional to take her shortness of breath seriously after an emergency C-section, as detailed in a 2018 feature in *Vogue*.[4] She eventually had life-saving surgery, but if someone had taken her concerns and symptoms to heart, they may have caught her pulmonary embolism in time before having to perform the drastic procedure she needed.[5]

IT ALL COMES DOWN TO HORMONES, INFLAMMATION, AND THE GUT

I felt a duty to figure out why I was so effing tired—not just for myself, but for so many other women who were overlooked by the health care system.

As I continued to do research, all signs pointed to a hormone imbalance. In fact, if you google some of these symptoms, you may come across a condition called "adrenal fatigue," or AF. Early in my medical training, I had studied the adrenal glands and their function — adrenaline, aldosterone, and cortisol production, often known as the "stress" hormones. But no one teaches about "adrenal fatigue" in medical school. That's because adrenal fatigue isn't recognized as an established health diagnosis (more on this in chapter 3).

But something about the concept intrigued me. Proponents of AF claim it is caused by chronic stress (check). Your adrenal glands are unable to keep pace with the demands of constant fight-or-flight alerts and thus are unable to keep pace producing the hormones needed to keep you going. It was a catch-all term that sounded really good on paper (or on-screen, in my case).

But even though adrenal fatigue wasn't in the medical literature, I *knew* something was off with my hormones — why else would I be tired all the time? So I continued to do research. What I found out made absolute sense: "Adrenal fatigue" did not exist, but these symptoms *did*. However, it was different than so-called adrenal fatigue — it was a full-on hormonal imbalance. As I upped the ante on my research on nutrition, the gut, and hormonal imbalances, I began to piece together a diet plan that could combat this fatigue.

Once again, I became my own guinea pig and started blogging about my findings. I put my own theories to the test and developed dietary strategies to try to boost my energy. I gave myself a complete overhaul — a mental, a hormonal, and an inflammatory reset. It was certainly not without false starts, like the time I tried the lemon juice–cayenne cleanse (you know, in the name of science) and fell face-first on the New York City pavement. But eventually I struck gold. I found the right mix that created a hormonal balance and resulted in *energy* that I hadn't had in years — naturally.

And people noticed. At first, my family was shocked and appalled when I started turning down traditional favorite foods like roti (flatbread) and treats like kaju katli (sweet diamond-shaped desserts with ghee sugar and nuts). My aunts were speechless — quite possibly for the first time ever. "What kind of life is it without sweets and roti?!" Mom would ask, shaking her head. They couldn't understand why I would ever turn down these standbys, and they teased me for living on just "grass." But soon they all marveled at how much energy and strength I had — how I could run, go into my practice, ride bikes with my kids, and then work on my book or blog without ever tiring — and they stopped pushing the sweets and carbs on me.

Then, a few years ago, I went on a trip with some physician friends to Machu Picchu. I realized for the first time how my renewed energy levels really made a huge difference during the daily hikes. While everyone else would get tired and had to stop, I could keep on going, like the Energizer Bunny. I had energy like I hadn't had in years. My friends asked how the heck I wasn't huffing and puffing after our treks. Even our experienced Peruvian tour guide came up to me and asked, "Don't you feel tired!? In all my years of being a guide, I swear I haven't seen *anyone* do this hike so effortlessly — male or female!" *Wait, really?* I thought. *I am not even breaking a sweat.*

I realized I was on to something. And I feel the need as a doctor to share it with you.

THE ENERGY TRIFECTA

By now I'm sure you're wondering: What was this plan that made me feel so good? The reset I developed — what I like to call the WTF plan, as in *why the eff* was I so tired? — is based on a few underlying factors that I will explain in more detail throughout this book. But here's the short version: Our hormones, immune system, and gut are closely linked, and it's very common for them to tip out of balance. The key to boosting your energy (and solving other health issues, to boot) is bringing these three systems back into balance.

Hormones

We have many different hormones in our body that act as the body's signal system and regulate most of its basic functions. You may be familiar with some common hormones, like estrogen and cortisol (known as the stress hormone), but there are many more that perform a beautiful and complicated role in the body, keeping things running smoothly.

Think of the hormone system as a complex and interconnected hormonal highway, much like a big city's busy highway system. These hormones all respond to hormonal signals from the brain and are all constantly moving and changing, depending on what's happening with your other hormonal glands. Your hypothalamus is connected to your pituitary glands, which impact your thyroid, which in turn is connected to your adrenals and your ovaries or testes. And they all connect back to one another and the brain.

Everything is connected. If there is an accident near exit 63 on the Jersey Turnpike, traffic will back up for miles, with slowdowns lasting for hours. It's the same thing with our body.

The Immune System

The immune system is our body's defense against invaders like viruses and disease. When you fight the flu or the common cold, your immune system is at work. Like brave infantry, the cells of your immune system are triggered to fight any virus or bacteria messing with your system. After that inflammation response, the soldiers are supposed to go back to base and turn off the alarm. But in the modern world, for a myriad of reasons, they never get the signal that the emergency is over, or the threat keeps coming back in the form of foreign foods or toxins. This leads to what is called "negative chronic inflammation." This inflammation response sends signals to the brain and the rest of the body that there is a threat.

Gut Health

Gut health refers to the balance of microorganisms in the digestive tract. New research shows that our gut health plays a vital role in our overall health, affecting everything from our cravings to our moods to, of course, our energy levels.

Hormones and the gut have a symbiotic relationship. Hormones affect the gut; and, in turn, bacteria in the gut modulate and produce hormones. Gut bacteria not only create hormones, but they also help balance, or bind, excess hormones. When your digestive system is off, it can affect nutrient absorption, which causes malnourishment, and can lead to a number of chronic problems and symptoms, including acid reflux, indigestion, irritable bowel syndrome, and more.

These three systems work so closely together and are so key to our health that I call them the "energy trifecta" — if one is out of balance, it creates an overall imbalance that steals the energy you need to get through your busy day. And when you fix one system, the other two will improve. Once things are in balance, your energy levels will shoot up.

When you think about it, this makes sense: if your body is working so hard to right itself because one (or all) of these systems are unbalanced, it has little energy to do anything else. You feel drained. And not only are you feeling really tired, but you don't have enough resources to do other tasks to keep the body working at full capacity. When this happens at a sustained pace — when you are chronically stressed and tired — you can become susceptible to allergies and disease. This is the connection between inflammation, disease, and energy. We need to reset these systems, stabilize our hormones, and balance the energy trifecta to ward off infections and disease.

The trick to this is that most common hormonal imbalances are hard to diagnose, *but* they are easy to fix with lifestyle and dietary changes. The key is optimizing this energy trifecta. To do this, I combined a food plan that targets inflammation and hormonal imbalance with a type of intermittent fasting that improves gut health and strengthens the immune system. Along with overhauling my own diet, I prioritized sleep, changed my exercise routine, and practiced managing stress levels. And in the last several years, the emerging research on intermittent fasting, circadian rhythms, and gut health has backed my own experience with science.

I knew that if my plan worked for me, it could work for others. I thought about my patients who complained about the same symptoms I had struggled with: "Why can't I seem to get enough sleep?" or "I have absolutely no energy." They were tired, moody, and their sleep, well, was a mess. I started treating my patients with the WTF plan. One by one, they experienced renewed vitality they thought they had lost forever. Once I started using this integrative approach in my clinical practice, I knew that I needed to share it more widely, so I developed a wellness practice offering online coaching. I've since coached thousands of patients through my courses, virtual consults, and in-person exams. Through trial and error and lots of positive case studies, I have learned how to apply the new science to the busy schedules of modern women.

The results of this program have been nothing less than astonishing. I've seen women who were anxious, tired, and worn-out become renewed, empowered, and transformed. *Finally,* I thought. It has taken too long for the sisterhood to get some respect and get the answers they deserve! Our current medical system — the one I was trained in — has given us little advice on how to take care of our bodies so that we don't end up sick and exhausted. I mean, I was a double-board-certified MD who spent years doing research and I didn't even have the answers for myself! We need more tools to help us live our lives to the fullest and healthiest. I am here to give them to you.

QUIZ

You might be wondering how strong your energy trifecta is. Here is a quick and easy (but by no means exhaustive) self-check. Just answer the following five questions on a scale of 1 to 5:

1. How good is your energy? 5 = awesome, I can do whatever I want when I want; 1 = I am so exhausted DAY AND NIGHT.
2. How often do you have trouble with constipation, gas, reflux, diarrhea? 5 = I am as regular as they come; 1 = I feel like I am constantly having issues.

3. If you are still of childbearing age, how regular is your period? 5 = I could set my watch to the day; 1 = my period is so erratic I never know when to expect it.
4. How often do you come down with a cold and other viruses? 5 = I have yet to miss a day of work; 1 = I feel like I am always battling something!
5. How is your mood? 5 = life is good; 1 = I tear up at every commercial.

Done? If your number is 20 or below as a premenopausal woman or below 15 as a man or postmenopausal woman, you need to work on this trifecta. Welcome — this book is for you! If your total is above 20, well, you may have some secrets to tell us!

THE ABC'S OF THE WTF PLAN

The food you eat can have a transformative effect. Take your metabolism, for instance. The right diet can often help keep your metabolic hormones in balance.

You know those people who can eat whatever they want and not gain a pound? And then there are some people who just look at a potato chip and gain five pounds? What gives? This is usually chalked up to the fact that everybody's metabolism is different, as if metabolism is something you can't really change. Your metabolism may be hard to change, but it is regulated by hormones, and what you are eating may be causing those hormones to go out of whack, which in turn effs with your metabolism, making you want to throw your scale out the bathroom window.

The right foods can also mitigate the need for hormone supplements, what we docs call "exogenous" (generated from outside) hormones. Even healthy women and men who follow a traditional healthy diet may experience fatigue, weight gain, brain fog, sleep issues, you name it, but usually their doctor will dismiss their concerns if lab tests come out negative. If they go to an alternative medicine center, they may be prescribed many supplements as well as exogenous hormones for their specific problem.

But oftentimes, these same issues can be fixed with diet. (Please know that if you're currently on some kind of hormone or other medication, I am not recommending that you drop it cold turkey because of this book — always speak with your medical doctor before changing any medication or doses.) Eating the right hormone-balancing foods that are rich in fiber, taking probiotics, and drinking healing teas can help realign this fragile system.

Diet doesn't just help with hormones; it helps with gut health. We're only just beginning to discover how important the gut is to our health and wellness, and how essential a healthy gut is to a healthy immune system. A recent study showed that babies had certain bacteria in their gut that "talked" to the immune system, telling it to tolerate foods like eggs or blueberries, indicating for the first time how early this connection between the immune system and gut bacteria is made.[6] When the immune system is just forming, it starts to makes decisions on what it considers good to pass along or foreign to reject, and this is when it develops food allergies (where the body deems the food as foreign). How food allergies are formed gives us a good insight on how the gut and immune system talk to each other in general — and just how early this connection is made. Further, it shows that our immune system and gut bacteria are in constant conversation all our lives, deciding which food to attack (e.g., if you had an allergy to peanuts) or which to tolerate (like greens and other vegetables) among thousands of other decisions. It starts from inside the womb and continues for our entire lifetime. The communication system between the gut, immune system, and the brain is my jam.

But this is only part of the story. I also found that *when* you eat is important to your overall health. Our bodies are made to run perfectly and work and rest right on time. We should take better advantage of our natural circadian rhythm — that internal clock that regulates the sleep-wake cycle and repeats roughly every 24 hours — to maximize our body's own resources. Eating according to the circadian rhythm will achieve better hormonal balance and pro-motes long-term health.

Now, you may have heard a lot about intermittent fasting because, well, it seems like everyone — your trainer, your child's teacher, heck, even your dentist — is trying it. Intermittent fasting is when you eat all of your food for the day within a specific window of time, often a 10-hour window (such as 10 a.m. to 8 p.m.) or an 8-hour window (such as 12 p.m. to 8 p.m.). Sometimes it means limiting your food to one meal a day. There are a lot of different variations, some better than others. My program — what I like to call circadian fasting — is different than a typical intermittent fasting diet because it works in sync with your body's natural clock. Since no one person is the same, and some schedules are more accommodating of circadian fasting than others, I will also provide creative solutions to work with your unique needs.

Managing stress is also a key component to keeping our system working properly. Daily assaults of stress can affect every part of the body, and the body-mind connection cannot be overstated. Stress hinders our sleep. It makes us distracted. Everyone has stress, and some stress is good for our body — but excessive stress, which re-leases too much cortisol, will totally zap your energy. The WTF plan will help balance stress in a couple of different ways — from the foods you eat to a few exercises that will help alleviate stress by strengthen-ing the mind-body connection that conventional medicine tends to overlook. (Namaste, bitches.)

HOW TO USE THIS BOOK

If you picked up this book, odds are you have been asking yourself the same question: *Why am I so effing tired?* You may feel tired from the time you get out of bed and set your feet on the floor to when you put your head back down on your pillow. Maybe you feel so bloated that you don't dare try on that bathing suit, too harried to find the eyeglasses that are sitting on top of your head, and so unfocused that you can't even read your favorite magazine. Are you ready for a reset that has been tested by not only me but thousands of other women — including Katie, whose sleep has improved so much that she is no longer counting sheep in her head — who can finally say they have won their fight with fatigue?

In this book, I will provide groundbreaking information on how the energy trifecta works, what happens when it doesn't, and what to do about it. You may notice similar solutions for each prong of the energy trifecta — diet, circadian fasting, stress reduction, sleep. This shows just how interconnected the three systems are, and how essential it is to address each of them — hormones, gut, immune system — at the same time. I'll show the important interplay of the mind-body connection and lay out a sensible, easy-to-follow two-week plan with the goal to align your gut health with your internal clock, which will in turn balance out your hormones and, most noticeably, make your energy skyrocket.

I make the plan flexible so that you can follow it to a T or make it fit your own goals and schedule. I will also provide information on how to integrate the plan into a more long-term program that fits your lifestyle. The diet is predominantly plant-based, as well as gluten-free and dairy-free, but you can certainly add meat, wheat, and dairy if you can tolerate them. (I just ask that you make high-quality choices, meaning read your labels and buy food that's as fresh and organic as possible.) My rule of thumb: follow 90 percent of my plan, leaving about 10 percent wiggle room for your own tastes.

The WTF plan has a three-pronged approach:

- *What You Eat:* Up your fiber-rich, *pre*biotic vegetables with plant-based recipes. We'll focus on prebiotic vegetables, such as artichokes, leeks, garlic, and asparagus, and cruciferous vegetables, such as bok choy, broccoli, brussels sprouts, cauliflower, and cabbage. Eating 6–8 servings a day will have a tremendous positive impact on your hormonal levels.

- *When You Eat:* By doing intermittent fasting in conjunction with our natural internal clocks (what I call circadian fasting), you'll revamp your energy.
- *Ease Your Stress:* Do simple exercises, get outside, turn off tech, and drink teas that ease anxiety. And sleep. Sleep is key to improving any type of previous hormonal blockage or imbalance. In a recent study published in the journal *Sleep*, people who only got six hours of sleep a night for two weeks started to function as poorly as those who stayed up two full nights without sleep.[7] Translation? Getting six hours of sleep or less is nearly as bad as getting none at all. Sleep loss impacts your cognition, your immune system, your energy, and your gut health. It can even affect your DNA. Sleep loss leads to epigenetic changes (changes that modify your cells' ability to read your genes) that can result in faster aging and reduced longevity. So for the sake of your genes, your gut, and your brain, figure out a way to sleep seven to nine hours most nights, and ideally go to bed before 11 p.m. I know sleep doesn't come easy to most people, and two to three nights a week of reduced sleep may not be too harmful. (Full disclosure: on average, I don't get my full night's sleep two days a week, and I haven't suffered for it.) But if you're someone who consistently gets less than six hours of sleep a night, consider it a New Year's resolution to get more sleep, no matter what time of year it is.

Plus, to help you in the plan, you will need to consider the following:

- *Exercise:* Be mindful of the type of exercise you are doing. If you work a very stressful job and lead an equally stressful life, limit your stressful workouts (such as HIIT or CrossFit) to three times a week. And remember, walking 8,000–12,000 steps is a really simple way to incorporate exercise into your everyday routine (just try to do it outside in nature as much as possible). Being easy on your body is best when trying to regulate any type of hormonal imbalance.

- *Supplements:* Although I discourage you from taking supplements that anyone promises will relieve you of any "adrenal fatigue" symptoms (or any hormonal imbalance for that matter), do consider taking well-studied natural supplements that are beneficial for your overall health picture, such as vitamin D and omega-3 and possibly adaptogens (herbal supplements that balance hormones naturally) like ashwagandha, amla berry, and rhodiola. I'll give you lots of guidance about what to take and how in chapters 7 and 8.

By learning how to access this energy trifecta, you will certainly feel better. And you will see change quickly: through advanced genome sequencing technology, we now know there are 100 trillion microbes in our body, the bulk of which lives in our gut—what's known as our microbiome. These microbes have their own DNA (about 3.3 million just in our gut), which greatly surpasses all of our entire body's DNA (23,000). Sort of mind-blowing when you think about it: you are really just a vessel in which these microbes live. But existential thoughts aside, studies show that this crowded microbiome can change quickly—in as little as three days![8] But while you can feel better and have more energy in such a short time, I want you to think of this as a lifestyle change rather than a quick fix. This isn't the kind of plan you do for two weeks and then you go back to your old ways (like a typical diet). In fact, the biggest problem with many diets is that they aren't sustainable. You white-knuckle it through the two-week or 30-day plan, until you can't anymore. And when you inevitably go back to eating normally, the problems return. So you then white-knuckle it through 30 more days. And the cycle repeats. Don't get me wrong, many thousands of people have benefited from popular diet plans. It's just that I want you to have consistency in a plan that is easy to manage over the long run—over years, even decades.

On the WTF plan, the magic happens after just two weeks. After two weeks, you'll ignite the real, life-changing benefits, and you will truly feel energy come surging back. But I don't want you to stop there. My plan walks you through twelve weeks total, focusing on the crucial first two weeks, and I promise that the longer you do the plan, the more you will get out of it. Along the way, I provide tips, alternatives, and variations so that you can personalize this plan to your needs and maximize its benefits. Whether it's tailoring the gut rest to your time schedule or adjusting foods that you prefer, this plan is for *you* and designed to last for as long as you want. I don't want you to just have increased energy for two weeks. What's the point of that? What if you could have that energy for a year, five years, ten? The rest of your life? That sounds like a good plan to me.

And a good plan always starts with due diligence. As a doctor, I know how important it is for my patients to consult with me before taking on any health plan; so remember to talk your own doctor before doing so. This book has my suggestions for a more energized life, not to be considered a substitution for medical advice, so check with your provider to make sure it's right for you and for any medical condition you may have. You want to get the thumbs-up before proceeding (and who knows, maybe he or she will want to try it too!).

So my hope is that this book becomes a crucial resource in helping you on a lifelong journey to a *revitalized* and healthy body, with *sustainable* energy, better focus, less bloat, and improved command of your daily stresses. (Hey, I never said I could completely rid you of your stress, but I can help you learn to manage it better.)

Ready to not feel so effing tired anymore? Read on.

1

What *Are* Hormones, Anyway?

IT WAS A HOT AND SWEATY MONDAY when I entered my office and saw Rita, a beautiful, dark-haired woman in her forties, sitting patiently in the waiting room. She was one of the few women whom I see in both my allergy/immunology practice as well as my wellness practice. We didn't have an appointment, but she was so sweet I didn't mind squeezing her in. I had time before my first appointment of the day, so I had her follow me into my office, where she had barely sat down before bursting into tears.

"Dr. Shah, I feel like something is wrong with me. I feel so emotional *all the time*. Half the time I want to kill my husband for the smallest infraction, then other times, I am crying like a baby, like right now. I have been back at work only for a few months after having my second child, but I am finding all of it really exhausting, and I am just always tired. Can you give me something to take to make me feel better?"

If only it were that simple! I had treated Rita for asthma for years, and from time to time she had some fatigue, bloating, and brain fog that pointed to a hormonal problem, too. But her lab work had always come back normal. But now, Rita's fatigue and mood instability were practically screaming hormonal imbalance. I assured Rita that I would help her, and my first step was to rule out any medical abnormalities by testing. Once those came back normal, we dove deep into hormones. This is what I told her.

MEET YOUR HORMONES

If you're like Rita — and like I was several years ago — you are probably thinking, *What the eff do hormones have to do with my fatigue?* Good question! Once I understood this connection, I was able to better understand my symptoms. I think you will, too.

But first, what exactly *are* hormones? When you think of the term, what's the first thing that comes to mind? A boy-crazy preteen who wears all black to match her angsty mood? Or the menopausal woman hoping she doesn't get a dreaded hot flash in the middle of her important meeting? Hormones get a bad rap — we only seem to think of them in the extremes of their functions, either at the height of puberty or at the decline of fertility. But that is only a fraction of what hormones do.

To better appreciate what can go wrong with our hormones, first we need to unpack what they are and what they do. And I should add the caveat here that the study of hormones is a young and imperfect science that's just a little over a hundred years old. While a lot has been discovered in that time, much remains a mystery. And what we *do* know is very, very complex. I will try to keep it as simple as possible while arming you with the right information to better understand how hormones work and how this information can help fix what's ailing you. I can tell you that even hormone experts admit that the constellation of symptoms that Rita and I had were common but hard to explain and treat.

So here's what we understand so far: The hypothalamic-pituitary-adrenal axis (HPA, for short) is a complex system that intertwines the central nervous system and the hormones, traditionally called the endocrine system. Hormones are chemical messengers, or communicators, produced mostly by specialized glands (and also by fat cells) located throughout our body—namely, the thyroid, adrenal glands, pituitary glands, pancreas, ovaries, and testes. Hormones are made of cholesterol, peptides, and/or amino acids. It's safe to say that hormones help control and regulate pretty much all of the body's complex activities, fluctuating throughout the day according to the body's needs. From the moment our alarm goes off in the morning, a shot of cortisol helps us wake up, and at night melatonin helps us relax and snuggle in for a restful sleep.

⁂

In fact, hormones are true rock stars when it comes to your body and your health, because they play a role in, well, pretty much everything and are responsible for our ability to operate day in, day out. Our hormones regulate most of our body's processes, from our metabolism and appetite to our heart rate, sleep cycles, reproductive and sexual functions, growth and development, mood and stress levels, and even our body temperature.

From what we now know, our brain orchestrates the signals on how and when hormones are released. They then travel through the body via the bloodstream, which acts much like a highway, helping our hormones to get to where they need to go. Once they arrive at their destination, they pass on messages to our organs and tissues by binding to specific target cells through receptors on the outside of the cell. Similar to a car parking in a garage, when the hormone and receptor bind, the cell or tissue snaps into action and performs its function. In fact, the word "hormone" comes from the Greek *hormōn*—"to set in motion." The crazy thing is that it doesn't end there. Hormones deliver the signal and then get feedback from the organ. This feedback signal turns around and gives the brain a message to adjust, stop, or increase its production of that specific hormone.

When our hormones are in balance, they keep us running smoothly, like a finely oiled machine, telling our organs what to do and when to do it. When they function well, we function well. It's that simple. But when there is too much or too little of a hormone in the bloodstream, that's when hormonal imbalances happen, and that's when we can get into trouble.

Even the smallest teeter of the delicate hormonal balance — what is more accurately called the hormonal axis — can put our whole system out of whack. When hormones are not in balance, that's when we notice it. We feel sluggish, distracted, or constantly stressed and, worse, if left untreated, hormonal imbalance can lead to chronic conditions, weight gain, and disease. For instance, a hormone released from the hypothalamus in the brain, the gonadotropin hormone-releasing hormone (GnRH), coordinates with our hypothalamic-pituitary-adrenal axis, so there is a strong link between hormonal imbalance and GnRH pulse disturbance: When your body is working well, this pulse runs smoothly, but when there is a lot of stress on the body — say, from exercise, fasting, outside events, or just plain bad eating — all of that stress can disturb the GnRH pulse, which in turn can cause a domino effect of hormonal imbalance throughout the body. (We also know that GnRH is heavily influenced by the circadian rhythm, but more on this later.)

What's more, since the bloodstream carries some fifty different hormones (I am convinced there are many more that have yet to be discovered) throughout the body in a pretty complicated process, one hormonal imbalance can affect other hormones. How? All of our hormones travel this busy highway, complete with on-ramps and exits; all respond to hormonal signals from the brain; and all are constantly moving and changing lanes depending on what's happening with our other hormonal glands. Everything depends on that highway running smoothly, with traffic flowing. When it's working correctly, it's flawless — we just go on with our busy lives. We've got game. But when something happens to cause a bottleneck or an accident, it throws off our whole system because it impacts everything on this highway. And we will feel it, usually in how it depletes our energy and makes us just want to take a nap (or two). That's because the body is working overtime to correct the imbalance, diverting our energy to that immediate need, making us tired, run-down, cranky, out of it, and off our game. And if the entire system is affected for too

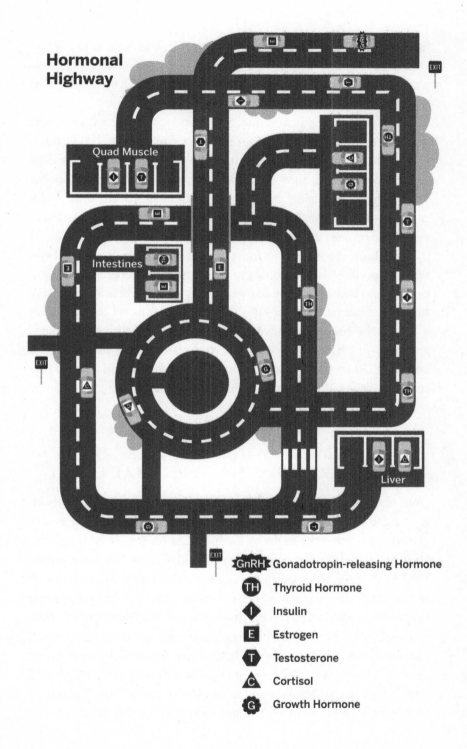

Hormonal Highway

GnRH — Gonadotropin-releasing Hormone

TH — Thyroid Hormone

I — Insulin

E — Estrogen

T — Testosterone

C — Cortisol

G — Growth Hormone

long, and we don't do anything to correct it, our overall health will suffer. By the time you go to a doctor to find out why you feel this way, a true diagnosis can be hard as it is often difficult to pinpoint the original culprit.

In traditional medical training, future doctors don't learn about the connection between this hormonal axis and energy levels, but it can be the key to reigniting our vitality. And even if your doctor does see the connection, they often isolate one hormone imbalance for your fatigue — ignoring the tethered relationship of the entire hormone system and possibly missing the fact that there are most likely several hormones at play.

Let's look at some of the most pivotal parts of the hormonal system, especially when it comes to producing and retaining your energy levels, and what happens when they get off track. While many hormones can become off-kilter, we'll concentrate on those that really suck the energy out of you and cause you to feel sluggish, foggy, and, *ugh, just not yourself.* Cortisol and estrogen are the two most common culprits in women, but we'll also cover insulin and the thyroid hormones since they play a big part in our vitality, too.

THE MASTER GLANDS (AKA THE PITUITARY AND THE HYPOTHALAMUS)

Both the pea-sized pituitary gland and the equally tiny hypothalamus are located near the base of the brain and are considered master glands — or, using the highway analogy, the on-ramps, as they kick-start most of the hormones you are familiar with. You have probably heard of human growth hormone (HGH) from the news — often called the "fountain of youth hormone," it's a naturally occurring hormone controlled by the pituitary gland that helps in growth (obviously) and in the healing process, but it's the synthetic version that some athletes take to amp up their performance (and then get in trouble if they get caught). (More on the naturally occurring HGH later.) The hypothalamus, which sits above the pituitary gland, is where the highway of hormone signals starts — it also decides to decrease or increase the flow in case of a traffic jam or accidents, to continue the metaphor. When there is a hormonal imbalance, it's not usually from one organ like the thyroid; instead it's usually a traffic pileup in the area of the thyroid. This will affect all the other hormones and feedback systems.

In addition, the pituitary gland produces hormones in its two distinct areas, the anterior lobe and the posterior lobe. The anterior lobe secretes six main hormones, and human growth hormone is the rock star of them all: integral to the body's physical development, it is responsible for making you tall and muscular like your aunt Sherri or petite like your aunt Sue. It's released at night and repairs the skin, gut, and muscles. They don't call 11 p.m. "beauty hour" for nothing —it's the time when you release growth hormone. You also get another little burst in the early morning. This plays a big part in making you tall or short, apple- or pear-shaped, old- or young-looking; it's not just your genes. The growth hormone also determines if an injury heals or not.

The pituitary also produces the thyroid-stimulating hormone, which stimulates the production of T3 and T4, which are important in regulating your body's temperature, metabolism, and heart rate. (Of course, these are also key to your energy levels — in fact, most doctors will run some sort of thyroid test for patients who complain of fatigue, since it's known for playing a role in energy levels and metabolism.) The posterior lobe of the pituitary releases only two hormones: an antidiuretic hormone, which regulates the amount of water excreted by the kidneys, making sure our body is well hydrated, and oxytocin.

Oxytocin and other brain hormones can pack a powerful punch in helping offset important imbalances in the rest of the body. For instance, feeling stressed? The hypothalamus produces the feel-good brain hormone oxytocin, which is called the "love hormone" since it plays a role in social bonding, childbirth, mother-child attachment, and intimacy. ("Love, lust, and labor," baby.) It also produces dopamine, which is released when you do things that make you feel warm and fuzzy, such as cuddling your dog, playing with your kids, listening to your favorite music, or even just performing a few breathing techniques.[1] In times of stress, these brain hormones can be called up and released as a great counterbalance to cortisol. (We'll talk later in the book about how to best harness these hormones to our advantage and increase energy levels.)

When our bodies are functioning correctly (good traffic flow, no accidents, no need for GPS), the hypothalamus talks to the pituitary, which is about the size of a pea, and in turn the pituitary produces hormones to direct other glands to produce *their* hormones. This creates a domino effect of reactions.

For instance, let's say you have to give a speech and you are anxious about it ... I bring this up because I still get nervous when I speak in public, no matter how many times I have done it. Here's what happens in my body as I walk up to the podium: The hypothalamus releases the corticotropin-releasing hormone (CRH), which in turn signals the pituitary gland to release its hormones to tell the adrenal glands to release their fight-or-flight hormones, that is, cortisol. Hello, now my palms are sweaty and, oh, look at that, my heart is racing, my breathing is fast, and my brain is hyper-focused. Don't bother asking me any complicated questions — the brain cannot handle complex tasks during this chain reaction. When the adrenals have done their duty (i.e., I am done with my speech), they will then send communication back that there are enough adrenal hormones available for the job and the cycle can end. This is an example of your hormones working properly. (If you are nervous about public speaking like I am, I bet just reading this paragraph triggered a little release of CRH to the pituitary and on to the adrenals — it's that fast!)

Pituitary Issues

Unlike most of the endocrine system, which (as you will read) can be restored to balance primarily by dietary and lifestyle choices, any sort of hormonal dysfunction in the pituitary gland is usually caused by disease (such as a tumor) and cannot be fixed by diet or lifestyle. Similarly, the hypothalamus can stop working too, but that is also likely triggered by a brain injury or tumor.[2] So any malfunction with the pituitary gland or hypothalamus likely means that medical intervention will be needed; diet and lifestyle changes can't help there.

THE THYROID HORMONE

Jennifer was a 35-year-old lawyer who recently came to me for food allergies.

"Dr. Shah, my skin is soooooo dry, like alligator skin. And my husband complains about my feet being ice blocks under the bedcovers. It's true my hands and feet are always cold. What the heck?" I questioned her more about her symptoms: she also had fatigue, a profound fatigue that she never had before. I decided to check her thyroid hormones along with some other blood work, and, lo and behold, her lab work showed that she had low levels of a thyroid hormone called "free T4." In her case, her fatigue was stemming from this one hormonal imbalance (just to be clear: this is not always the case).

So what is the thyroid, which gave Jennifer so much grief? The butterfly-shaped thyroid is located at the base of the neck on both sides. The hormones released here do a lot of the work to regulate your energy and your metabolism, and they also have a hand in heart function, digestion, brain development, mood, and bone health. You may have heard that iodine is important for a well-balanced thyroid, which is true, but thyroid health depends on a good diet as well. The thyroid hormone is made by taking iodine (from food) and combining it with the amino acid tyrosine to make triiodothyronine (T3) and thyroxine (T4), which are then released into the bloodstream and transported throughout the body, where they help with all the functions stated above — but when they aren't working properly, they just may be the reason you are dragging all the time.

How, exactly? Well, let's put it all together: In the simplest case (which is not that simple, I admit), the hypothalamus releases TRH (thyrotropin-releasing hormone), which signals the pituitary to release TSH (thyroid-stimulating hormone) to tell the thyroid gland to produce more T4. So when T4 levels are low in the blood, the pituitary gland releases more TSH to tell the thyroid gland to produce more thyroid hormones. So in Jennifer's case, we saw a high TSH and low T4, which let us know her thyroid function was low, the telltale cause of her fatigue. She had hypothyroidism, and I put her on my plan as well as thyroid replacement therapy, and she was shocked by how much better she felt in just a matter of weeks.

But there are other types of thyroid problems that don't come up with conventional testing. Here are a few questions that you can use to tell if your thyroid is off:

- Is the outer third of your eyebrows sparse?
- Do you have sudden weight gain?
- Do you have a hoarse voice?
- Are you puffier than usual?
- Do you have fatigue? (Of course you do — you are reading this book!)

Thyroid Issues

There are several hormones intimately connected to energy and metabolism produced by the thyroid. We have discussed triiodothyronine (T3) and thyroxine (T4), which work together as a kind of thermostat for the body's inner system. When working as it should, the thyroid keeps your metabolism running like a purring engine — you have a spring in your step and can think on your feet. When it's not running properly, a host of problems ensue. And it's very common, unfortunately: one in eight women will develop a thyroid condition in their lifetime.

Release too much of T3 and T4, and you have a hyperthyroid, a body on overdrive with irritability and sleep issues. If too low of a release, you have hypothyroidism, which surfaces as low metabolism, weight gain, fatigue, and sensitivity to the cold (I'm talking about those who wear three sweaters in 80-degree weather). So, it is important that T3 and T4 levels are neither too high nor too low. Two glands in the brain — the hypothalamus and the pituitary — communicate to maintain T3 and T4 balance.

Hypothyroidism (Underactive Thyroid) and/or Hashimoto's Disease

Sadly, too many thyroid conditions go undiagnosed because of inconclusive tests — or because they're not tested for at all. It depends on whom you talk to, but I would say that most people don't have symptoms. One study found that 73 percent of hypothyroid patients and 68 percent of hyperthyroid patients had elevated thyroid antibodies (indicating that the body's immune system is attacking the thyroid) prior to the onset of thyroid dysfunction.[3] Another study reports that 50 percent of patients, mostly women, have thyroid nodules (growths).[4] If there are symptoms, they include a sensitivity to cold (much like my patient Jennifer), constipation, fatigue, weight gain, and muscle weakness. Low thyroid action can also cause depression; as much as 15–20 percent of depression sufferers have been shown to have a hypothyroid.[5] If you have been diagnosed with hypothyroidism, it was most likely caused by Hashimoto's disease, an autoimmune condition, and you will need to be put on medication. Note, when you put out the fire in your gut and the immune system, you may see your thyroid health improve and symptoms subside or go away. However, I don't recommend changing or stopping medication, especially without consulting your doctor.

What Is Hashimoto's Disease?

Hashimoto's is an autoimmune disease whereby your immune system attacks the thyroid. The disease progresses slowly and often causes hypothyroidism, but because its symptoms are similar to hypothyroidism, it is hard to diagnose. The cause is unknown, but there are a few factors that play a role, such as genetics, gender (women are more likely to develop the disease), and age (the disease is commonly seen in middle age, although it can occur at any age).

Telltale Signs of Hypothyroidism

- Slow heartbeat
- Cold hands and feet
- Puffy face
- Cold intolerance
- Weight gain
- Brittle nails and dry skin and hair
- Enlarged thyroid
- Heavy menstrual periods
- Fluid retention
- Bowel movements less than once a day
- Lethargy/fatigue especially in the morning
- Depression
- Forgetfulness

Hyperthyroid

Under the influence of the thyroid-stimulating hormone (TSH), the thyroid can also produce too much T3 and T4, making you irritable and wired — you may even experience heart palpitations. It can also hasten your body's metabolism, causing weight loss. In the long term, hyperthyroidism can cause serious problems with the heart, bones, muscles, menstrual cycle, and fertility. Only 1.2 percent of people get this, women more than men, but rates increase as we grow older.[6] And recent studies have shown that low microbial diversity in the gut can help put the thyroid on overdrive[7] (something we will get to later in this chapter, and again in chapter 5).

Telltale Signs of Hyperthyroidism

- General tiredness
- Muscle weakness

- Lump in the neck from enlarged thyroid
- Weight loss
- Irritability
- Frequent bowel movements
- Hair loss
- Sweating and warm, sweaty palms
- Heat intolerance
- Rapid heartbeat
- Soft nails
- Difficulty sleeping
- Very light periods

If you do suspect a thyroid issue, you can log onto thyroid.org and find a board-certified endocrinologist in your area.

THE PANCREATIC HORMONES

I have a lot of personal experience with the major hormone of the pancreas (i.e., insulin) because of my strong family history of type 2 diabetes. (Type 1 diabetes is an autoimmune disease where the body can't produce insulin, and type 2 is a metabolic condition mostly brought on by lifestyle and diet, with a genetic component, and is caused by being insulin resistant.) As you may know, a lot of people with diabetes have a problem with their pancreas not making enough of the hormone insulin. Did you know that one of the main presentations of diabetes is fatigue?

Located in the abdomen, behind the stomach, the pancreas plays an essential role in converting the food we eat into fuel for the body's cells. It produces the hormone insulin, which helps cells function by "feeding" them blood sugar for energy. How this is done is another example of the body's amazing natural orchestration: Let's say you have a pancake. The carbohydrates are digested and broken down into glucose and passed into the bloodstream. The pancreas detects the release of glucose and will start to secrete its main hormone, insulin, into the circulatory system to collect the glucose and deliver it to your cells for energy. (If you drink a milkshake along with this potato pancake, the insulin release would be much greater because of all the sugar.) The pancreas's second main hormone, glucagon, helps insulin by working as an opposing force, getting your cells to release glucose.

If insulin becomes imbalanced, meaning constant sugar spikes that make insulin less responsive, it can negatively impact your metabolism and the ability to maintain a healthy weight. For example, if you constantly eat foods that are too sugary, your insulin levels will remain high for an extended period of time. This will cause insulin resistance, which is when too much insulin is needed to do the same job that it used to do and it gets "tired" and cannot effectively transport glucose from the blood into cells any longer. The cells "resist" taking in glucose, and therefore blood glucose remains elevated, so as a "reflex" the pancreas pumps out more insulin. (We'll get into this more below.)

The importance of insulin cannot be overstated: high insulin levels and high glucose can cause a host of issues, like weight gain, some cancers, heart disease, and type 2 diabetes — just like my dad and other relatives had. Many people with both types of diabetes have a problem with their pancreas not making enough insulin. Some experts believe that some people are genetically susceptible to type 2 diabetes. Even if you don't have diabetes, knowing about the pancreatic hormones is important in thinking about a healthy diet — so you don't raise your risk of getting diabetes.

What Is Insulin Resistance?

Insulin is a growth hormone. If, after eating a meal, your insulin response is working correctly, your pancreas will begin to release insulin into your bloodstream, which will then travel to your cells to hand off glucose and will stop releasing it when it receives signals to stop. Too much insulin can create a condition known as "insulin resistance." How does this happen exactly? When you eat a sugary meal, your insulin levels shoot up, and if you consistently eat sugary meals, day after day, the pancreas will continue to produce too much insulin. Picture this scenario as a mother (insulin) who yells at her small child (our cells) morning and night. After a while, the child starts to ignore the yelling, and the receptor cells don't take in the insulin that they should, or they "resist."

Unfortunately, the pancreas continues to make more insulin to try to make up for the resistance, but eventually the production can't keep up the pace and slows down. As the pancreatic beta cells get burned out (simply called "beta burnout")[8] and not enough insulin is made, blood sugars will start to rise above normal. Welcome to prediabetes. If the above-normal sugars continue for a good amount of time, the condition will progress into type 2 diabetes. Sadly, if there are too many beta cells damaged, it can become very difficult to reverse the condition.

While insulin resistance is well known as a stepping-stone to prediabetes and diabetes, it can also lead to other serious conditions, including heart disease, Alzheimer's, depression, high blood pressure, and high cholesterol. The best way to treat this "pre"-prediabetes condition is through — you guessed it — lifestyle and dietary changes.

What's more, insulin resistance brings with it a huge problem for younger women: studies indicate that it can be the root cause of polycystic ovary syndrome (PCOS). While the connection has been made,[9] researchers still aren't quite sure *why*. For now we just know that for younger women with insulin issues, it results in PCOS; for older women, it's heart disease. On a recent trip to New Delhi, India, for a wellness conference, I met so many young women who exhibited a cascade of symptoms, such as weight gain, problems with fertility, acne, and PCOS. There was one sweet 26-year-old in particular, Pooja, who pulled me aside and told me of her issues with her weight, her period irregularity, and her breakouts.

"I am a grown woman — why do I still get zits?!" she asked me.

I assured her she was not alone. "Believe it or not, adult acne is on the rise, primarily because of the increase of sugar and simple carbs in our diet." We talked about what she ate, and I gave her some quick tips on how to treat her likely insulin issue and assured her that she would soon see improvement if she changed her diet.

Telltale Signs of Insulin Resistance

- Always hungry and/or thirsty
- Tingling in hands or feet
- General fatigue
- Obesity
- High blood pressure, high cholesterol

Low insulin can be another culprit. With people who make little insulin, glucose levels rise and the cells cannot take in glucose for energy, and other sources of energy (such as fat and muscle) are needed to provide this energy. This makes the body tired and can cause weight loss.

ADRENAL HORMONES

Sherri first came to see me because a naturopath told her that she had "adrenal fatigue."

"What does that even mean?" she asked me.

"Well," I answered, "it's complicated. But first, you should know what the adrenals are and why they are such a hot topic when it comes to feeling tired. Many people believe that adrenal fatigue is the diagnosis when it's not." We'll discuss a little later about how the popular term "adrenal fatigue" is a misnomer, but first let's talk about how the adrenals work.

These triangular-shaped glands that sit atop each kidney are responsible for the mother lode of hormones, cortisol and adrenaline. Commonly known as the "fight-or-flight hormones," they help us in times of great stress. The body is naturally hard-wired to protect itself against assaults, and if it sees a perceived threat — like a huge bear or tiger baring its teeth — it will release cortisol and adrenaline to signal to the body to switch into survival mode, helping us run faster and protect ourselves.

While this was a great survival instinct thousands of years ago when we needed to outrun actual bears and tigers, it's not quite as helpful in today's world of constant stressors like work emails, traffic, and the daily grind. When our body receives a modern threat — like a looming deadline, an oncoming car, or a family emergency — the adrenals first release a sister hormone to cortisol, adrenaline (or epinephrine), which acts like a quick jolt of energy for the short term, giving us those telltale and immediate signs of stress, like a raised heart rate and heavy breathing. Then the adrenals release cortisol and norepinephrine (or noradrenaline) for a longer and more significant response to the threat. Once the danger is gone (the deadline is met, the crash is avoided, or the family emergency has resolved itself), your cortisol level should decrease, and other body reactions — like that feeling of your heart thumping out of your chest — should calm down as well. Just like when I finished giving that speech — my breath slowed, my hands stopped sweating, and I could think clearly again.

The problem occurs when the adrenal glands get overloaded, which, as you can imagine, is so common in today's stressful world. Too much consistent stress will mess with your system, period. Historically, cortisol saved our lives, helping us outrun that bear. But although today's attackers are different, our body's reaction is the same. Your body doesn't differentiate between the hungry bear and the nasty email that landed in your in-box, even though one is life-threatening and one is ... well, not pleasant, but not going to kill you. Because of this, your adrenal glands never have a chance to actually calm down — with constant threats, they get overloaded with all the stressors we live with, sort of like an overheated car. This was Sherri's issue — and it may be yours, too. Sherri and I worked together to identify the major stressors in her life and to figure out a healthier way to handle them with the WTF plan — as I explain later in chapter 8.

While cortisol is best known as the "stress hormone," it also manages a host of other functions, like helping the body better utilize carbohydrates, fats, and proteins; decreasing inflammation; keeping blood pressure stable; and normalizing our sleep cycles. It also helps the body manage its glycemic control, which is its ability to metabolize carbohydrates efficiently so that we don't experience peaks and valleys in blood sugar levels. When our cortisol goes out of whack, fatigue becomes a huge problem.

Cortisol Imbalance

No doubt if you are a high achiever (like many of my female patients), you are going to have cortisol issues. Cortisol is often considered the queen bee of hormonal balance — this adrenal hormone affects a wide range of functions throughout the body, such as regulating blood sugar, inflammation, the immune system, and, most important, our response to stress. It is also the most common imbalance in the twenty-first century, no doubt brought on by today's frenetic pace of work and home life.

On a normal day, cortisol fluctuations, referred to as the "cortisol curve" or the "circadian cortisol pattern," resemble a downward bell curve: you wake up and within 30 minutes your body produces its highest amounts of cortisol for the day, but cortisol production should gradually decrease and hit the lowest point at bedtime. When you get stressed out — by a difficult phone call, a crying child, a looming work deadline, or all three at once! — you make and release more cortisol. So much cortisol can be released on that highway that it can create a bottleneck — much like how a traffic jam forms when a busy three-lane highway needs to merge into one lane; everything slooooooooooows down, which in turn will create other hormonal slowdowns.

These "normal" stresses may be taking a toll on the brain in midlife, a recent study shows. Those who performed poorly on tests that assessed memory, organization, and focus had the highest levels of cortisol. Researchers also saw that the poor performance/high cortisol link was worse for women (although they couldn't determine if it was because women just had more stress than men or it just manifested in higher cortisol levels).[10] Can't find your phone or keys? Blame cortisol.

❧

If there is a traffic jam anywhere, and if the traffic is consistent (meaning your stress levels are always high and thus your body is constantly making excess cortisol), it can cause a cortisol imbalance, or "dysregulated" cortisol, as well as affect the levels of progesterone and estrogen. This can lead to a bunch of possible scenarios, discussed below.

High Cortisol

Bursts of cortisol production in reaction to stress are meant to be infrequent, intended to give us quick pops of energy that help get us through the most urgent hassles of the day (or outrun that hungry tiger). Then the spikes are supposed to stop, allowing our system to return to its normal state.

But today, many women, like myself before my accident, are constantly hitting that alarm button with daily, minute-by-minute insults to our stress levels. When there are persistently elevated levels of cortisol production over a long period of time, it can cause major upset throughout your body in the form of hypercortisolism, which in the long term can be detrimental to your overall health. A high cortisol imbalance is probably the most common of the hormone imbalances for women — in today's manic, chaotically busy world, it's surprising that we don't all have it!

When we have a stressful day — whether it's stress from diet or a lack of sleep or a host of emotional factors (where is that damn subway?), we end up making a lot of cortisol. And cortisol requires pregnenolone, which is often called the "mother hormone." There's a new theory about the role pregnenolone plays in hormone imbalance that's still being tested,[11] but it makes the most sense to me based on everything I've determined about hormones, energy, and stress. We have very limited levels of pregnenolone in our bodies, and it requires a lot of cellular energy to produce it, by converting cholesterol into pregnenolone. That means if you are really, really stressed, then a lot of energy will be used to make pregnenolone to in turn produce cortisol. All the energy will be channeled there instead of being channeled toward producing estrogen and testosterone and other hormones. This is called "pregnenolone steal" — pregnenolone is stealing valuable resources to make cortisol to the detriment of other hormones — and it can wreak havoc on your entire system.

My patient Sara is a perfect example of what this looks like in real life. Sara is a 45-year-old physician with three kids. When she first came to see me, she had a demanding home life that matched her demanding work life, and needless to say she felt burned out at both. She tried to make some self-improvements, reading articles that gave advice on increasing her energy, as many women do. She started getting up earlier to work out, thinking that exercise would give her more energy, and really the only time she could afford to do it was in the morning. So her alarm would go off at 4:30 a.m.(!), and she'd head off to some incredibly high-intensity class like CrossFit six days a week. Then on Sundays, instead of taking the day off, she did weights or some form of aerobics at home.

During the workweek, after her sweat sessions, she'd hurry home to get her kids off to school and her butt to work. The evenings were equally rushed as she'd race out of the office to get dinner on the table, put the kids to bed, and finally go to sleep at 11 p.m. Next day, repeat. She gave herself little time for any connection or mindfulness to herself and loved ones. She thought she was making positive changes to her life, but she was still feeling exhausted. When we met, she explained her daily routine to me, and a few things stood out immediately: she was raising her cortisol level *way* too many times a day, and she was not giving her body enough time to rest and recuperate.

The high-intensity workouts that Sara added to her daily routine can create a hormonal stress, or hormesis, which typically is great for building a stronger body. Each time you exercise, you are pushing your body to handle the stress a little bit more from the previous session, making it stronger for the next workout. Intense workouts are made this way to do exactly that, to make us stronger. But there must be recovery time. It's in the recovery that the muscles get stronger; if you don't take the time to recover and your body is in constant hormesis, it is not getting the benefits from the exercise — in fact, it becomes detrimental.

I recommended that Sara cut her morning workouts to two days a week, to allow herself four days to sleep in (hit the snooze button, go ahead!). I also told her to take 20-minute nature walks daily, so she was still being active, but not at such a high intensity that she was wiping herself out. (The nature walks were intentional since being outside in the natural environment is known to help decrease cortisol release.) We changed her diet from high sugar to high fiber, with an emphasis on probiotics to help the gut, and had her work in two days of circadian fasting. Within four *days* her energy was up, and within two months she lost weight, her cholesterol was lower, and she was sleeping better. She was amazed at her improvement. She, a doctor herself, had not heard hormones discussed in such a way before, and she was blown away by how a few simple changes could affect her health so markedly.

Telltale Signs of High Cortisol

- Wired but tired
- Feeling distracted
- Weight gain, particularly the midsection, aka "muffin top"
- Skin conditions like acne, eczema, and thin skin
- Sugar cravings
- Easy bruising

Sara showed classic signs of high cortisol, but high cortisol can also affect our digestive system and cause a host of conditions such as irritable bowel syndrome (we'll talk about the gut and cortisol a bit later in this chapter). Not only does cortisol increase your appetite, but it can also cause muscle and bone loss, and a decrease in sex drive. And there have been extensive studies showing that persistently high levels of cortisol can also cause abdominal fat. So bottom line: long-term cortisol spikes make us older, fatter, and more depressed than we should be. Um, no thanks.

If you are constantly in a state of panic, overworked, and frazzled, you are probably making too much cortisol. If you are feeding this stress by over-caffeinating and consuming too much sugar and omega-6 fats (found in fried foods, cured meats, and processed snacks like potato chips), you are only adding fuel to the fire. Similarly, simple carbs such as bread, cookies, cake, and so on act like sugar in the body and also affect glycemic control. Alcohol is another major culprit because it increases stress hormones just like cortisol —which is surprising (and a bummer for many of my patients!) since drinking alcohol is a common way that people try to deal with stress and anxiety. (But if you love your vino, don't worry, there's still room for the occasional glass of wine on the WTF plan.)

Drink a lot of caffeine? You're just pumping out these cortisol cars from the adrenal glands to all over the body, like the brain, muscles, and blood vessels. This cortisol is taking up all the lanes on the highway and blocking other hormones — like estrogen or progesterone — from getting to where they need to go, and you've got a traffic jam bigger than those on LA's 405. Sure, coffee gives you an energy surge, but too much will cause your heart rate and blood pressure to go up, with the result that you will get all jittery and more hyper than a teenager on the last day of school. Note: Some people can tolerate caffeine more than others depending on their genetic makeup. If you are one of those people, still limit your coffee intake from one to three cups.

Low Cortisol

This is often mislabeled as adrenal fatigue, adrenal burnout, and other similar misnomers in the media. Like elevated cortisol, this can cause you to feel exhausted and drained, like a car running on empty. It is actually common to develop low cortisol after a sustained amount of time dealing with high cortisol. Hypocortisolism, or low cortisol, is when your body is unable to produce enough cortisol, typically because it had been on overload for so long that it's tripping a fuse — the excessive demands overload the system, so all of a sudden it can't produce as much.

Prolonged low cortisol levels could also be an indication of a more serious problem in the pituitary or adrenal glands, perhaps caused by Addison's disease. Changes in your skin, like hyperpigmentation, or darkening, as well as muscle weakness, diarrhea or nausea, weight loss, and dizziness are all symptoms. This can be potentially life-threatening if not treated.

SEX HORMONES

Did you know that sex hormones — mainly estrogen and progesterone — are two key hormones that get imbalanced and often cause fatigue? I certainly didn't, at least not in the way we are talking about here. It's something that I learned on my own well after medical training.

Our sex hormones are very complex, responsible for many hormonal and physical changes that happen over the span of a lifetime, from puberty to pregnancy to menopause. The key hormones involved in sexual function include estrogen, testosterone, and progesterone, which all help in regulating reproductive function, sexual performance, libido, and even gender identification. The constant maturation of them makes them (like many relationships hatched by these very hormones) . . . so very complicated.

Sex hormones, especially in women, modulate so much of health and give women the superpower to create and support a human being. Because estrogen, progesterone, and testosterone are so interconnected with the rest of your body, it's no surprise that if we alter their delicate balance, we can experience a wide range of symptoms.

To better understand the female sex hormones, let's first revisit the angsty preteen. She will most likely hit the peak of puberty soon if she hasn't already, as most girls reach this milestone between the ages of 8 and 13. Once this happens, adrenal glands and ovaries will produce and release progesterone, estrogen, and testosterone into the blood. This sets off some obvious physical changes, like the sudden appearance of breasts, a growth spurt, armpit and pubic hair growth, and activated sweat glands (it's suddenly time to add bras, razors, and deodorant to the shopping list).

For girls, the hormone estrogen is especially key during puberty, as it is essential to normal cerebral growth and aids with breast, brain, vaginal, and ovarian development. Progesterone is a steroid hormone involved in the female menstrual cycle, as well as pregnancy, human fetal development, and more. A woman's first menstrual cycle occurs toward the end of puberty, often a full two years after the hormonal changes have begun (adding to the list tampons and pads, and maybe some Tylenol for the cramps).

The sex hormones also play a major role in pregnancy and childbirth — let's take our preteen and speed up her life. If and when she gets pregnant, her body will produce the hormone human chorionic gonadotropin (HCG), which prompts uterine growth to support the growing baby's immune system. The surge of HCG, estrogen, and progesterone causes classic pregnancy symptoms like nausea and vomiting. Along with another hormone, relaxin, progesterone facilitates the relaxing of uterine walls to accommodate the baby and helps loosen the pelvic ligaments to facilitate eventual vaginal birth (but it destabilizes hips and the spine in the process).

Now let's revisit the middle-aged woman petrified of hot flashes making an appearance at her important meeting. She is most likely experiencing perimenopause — the period in which levels of particular hormones decrease, or "sputter." Ovaries begin to make less estrogen and at menopause, which technically occurs 12 months after the last menstrual period, stop releasing eggs.

Men also have hormonal shifts as they reach puberty, which for them occurs between the ages of 9 and 14. Since most of you reading this book are women, I'll just touch on these male hormones: testosterone is the primary hormone for males that causes their reproductive organs to mature, their muscles and bones to grow, facial and pubic hair to appear, and voice to deepen. Testes develop, along with body hair and sweat gland activation (that gives way to loads and loads of smelly gym clothes). This sequence takes anywhere from two to five years: the hypothalamus secretes LSH, which stimulates the pituitary gland to secrete LH, which tells the testes to produce testosterone and FSH, which, in addition to testosterone, tells the testes to start producing sperm. Uh, more acronyms. Promise, we're mostly done. (Remember GnRH? Well, that helps release LSH and

FSH, so you can see that if GnRH isn't working correctly, then your reproductive organs won't, either.)

Both men and women have testosterone, though it's much higher in men. In males, the testes synthesize large amounts of testosterone. In females, the ovaries and the adrenal glands synthesize a much smaller amount. But in both men and women, this hormone is critical for maintaining ideal body composition, tissue repair, cholesterol balance, and brain, energy, and immune function.

Estrogen Imbalance

Estrogen is what makes us uniquely female, thank you very much, although males have a certain amount of the hormone as well. It's pivotal in our sexual development and, along with progesterone, regulates the entire reproductive system throughout our lives. It's hard to decide what level of estrogen is normal — this is widely different among women and the time of their cycle — what's more important is the *balance* of estrogen to progesterone. We should always strive to have both of them working together as a team. Otherwise we get a seesaw effect — if you have high estrogen, you'll have low levels of progesterone, and vice versa.

High Estrogen

When there is too much estrogen produced, the delicate balance will falter and cause estrogen dominance, which will make women gain weight (especially in our baby-bearing hip section, like Sara), feel tired, and — not surprisingly — suffer from a low libido. If you think you have this, you are not alone: up to 80 percent of women over 35 may be affected, although it's hard to diagnose.[12] Next to cortisol, this is the biggest imbalance for women and, like high cortisol, it will cause a heck of a lot of fatigue. And the most likely culprit? Our environment. Unfortunately, it's where we get a lot of impostors that like to mess with our system. These xenoestrogens, or "foreign" estrogen, are synthetic or natural compounds that mirror the molecular structure of estrogen. Many of these compounds are found in our everyday products — such as birth control, beauty products, plastics, and even some foods — and when they infiltrate our body, this can set off high estrogen symptoms. We can further complicate their effects by not doing enough to offset the imbalance, which can lead to more serious conditions like cancer and Hashimoto's (an autoimmune disease that attacks the thyroid).

The Pill

To pill or not to pill, that is the question, no? According to a 2012 US Department of Health and Human Services report, about two-thirds of American women of reproductive age use a form of contraception. Of those, about a third use the pill — about 10.6 million women.[13] For many, it has been a godsend either to avoid pregnancy or as a fail-safe for a multitude of health reasons — acne, aggressive PMS symptoms, and cancer prevention. But there are certainly downsides. After all, the pill is a cocktail of sex hormones that alters your body's homeostasis. So that's why many women can have a difficult time getting back to normal once they stop taking it. It can disrupt our natural hormone regulation, causing a condition called "post–birth control syndrome." In the months after getting off the pill, women can experience headaches, mood swings, acne, fertility issues, and irregular periods, among other symptoms.

It's a complicated discussion, one that can't be covered in a few paragraphs in this book, but there is a lot of fearmongering out there about what birth control pills can and cannot do to you. So, yes, the pill plays with your hormones, and doctors should be more careful in prescribing it. We want to be aware of these potential hormonal disruptions, but if you're in a situation where this is your cheapest, most accessible option for birth control, it's still a better option than nothing.

Telltale Signs of High Estrogen

- Exaggerated PMS symptoms such as heavy bleeding
- Extra weight, especially around the hips
- Bigger boobs
- Weepiness and moodiness
- Fatigue

Elevated estrogen can also lead to a higher BMI, irritability, depression, and carb cravings, (oh, hi, bread, where have you been all my life?). In the long term, high estrogen makes you more likely to develop breast tenderness, cysts, fibroids, endometriosis, and breast cancer. Low progesterone, which comes in tandem with high estrogen, can also be a problem, as it can be a side effect of high estrogen levels and can cause infertility, night sweats, sleeplessness, and irregular menstrual cycles.

Low Estrogen

While it is much more common to have too much estrogen, women can suffer from low estrogen production as well, which will cause your mood and libido to tank. Estrogen affects a wide range of the body's functions (e.g., bone development, menstrual regulation, and moods), and we can point to several causes of low estrogen levels. These include excessive exercise, thyroid conditions, and malnutrition, but the most common factor really has to do with age and where we are in our sexual life cycle. With perimenopause (in women over 40), estrogen naturally declines, and with menopause, estrogen is no longer being produced. Symptoms? All things we look forward to as we age (not): painful sex due to vaginal dryness, mood swings and depression, those telltale hot flashes, and breast tenderness.

Telltale Signs of Low Estrogen

- Low libido with matching low mood
- Lapses in memory and trouble concentrating
- Hot flashes
- Breast tenderness
- Bladder issues – either frequent UTIs or leaky bladder
- Missed periods

While cortisol, the thyroid, and estrogen are the three hormonal systems that are key to our energy levels, there are two other hormones that can also be important in keeping our energy levels to a maximum: testosterone and insulin.

Testosterone

While testosterone is typically thought of as only a male hormone, women make this hormone to a lesser degree in our ovaries and adrenals — and having it keeps our hair and skin healthy, makes us excited for sex, and gives us good muscle tone. It also helps with memory and focus, as well as keeping our energy up. So when levels are low, all these go to shit: we have thinning hair and dry skin; intercourse is painful because of dryness (not to mention loss of libido); and we can have a loss of muscle tone, depression, and general fatigue. Reasons for low production of testosterone in women have not been easy to uncover, but some doctors point to adrenal insufficiency, having an oophorectomy (the removal of the ovaries), oral estrogen therapy, and early menopause. But our own genetic makeup could affect the ability to produce the compounds DHEA and DHEA-S, both precursors to testosterone. Some women may also be deficient in enzymes that process these compounds into testosterone. (If it's not one thing, it's another!)

Telltale Signs of Low Testosterone

- Muscle weakness
- Bone loss
- Low libido
- Weight gain
- Fertility issues

THE GUT

The role the gut plays in our hormone health has been overlooked for years. The gut does a whole lot more than process our food, and it's now getting its due credit: recent studies have shown that there are millions of microbiota bacteria in your gut — that is, the micro-biome — and that gut bacteria are in constant communication with our immune system, signaling many of our hormones on what to do and what not to do.[14]

There is a *direct* connection between the gut microbiome, our hormones, and the brain center that controls our hormones (such as the hypothalamus). We'll get into this later in chapter 5, but new studies suggest that gut microbiota influence all of our hormones much more than we originally realized. Hormones — especially those created by the thyroid, as well as estrogen and cortisol — interact with the gut, which increases or decreases their levels. The gut can also help stabilize our metabolism, slow the aging process, and improve our moods.

There is a wealth of knowledge that is being discovered every day about how the gut affects our health, and I am particularly obsessed with this gut-hormone connection because I think it's the *key* to reclaiming our energy. There have been a few groundbreaking studies that indicate how the gut's microbiome affects our estrogen levels much more powerfully than we originally thought.[15] There's growing evidence that a group of microbes known as the "estrobolome," a big buzzword in the medical community, plays a significant role in metabolizing estrogen.

The estrobolome produces the enzyme beta-glucuronidase, which helps metabolize estrogen. When the gut microbiome is healthy, the estrobolome produces just the right amount of beta-glucuronidase to maintain estrogen homeostasis. However, when there is gut dysbiosis (or an imbalance), beta-glucuronidase goes out of whack, which in turn makes estrogen levels go haywire right along with it. And an imbalance among these bacteria can cause a host of issues like, *hello,* bloating, weight gain, and even acne, as well as the potential for developing estrogen-related diseases such as endometriosis, polycystic ovary syndrome, breast cancer, and prostate cancer.

Besides this newly discovered interaction between gut and hormones, the gut plays a major role in your appetite. It sets off tried-and-true alarm bells of hunger, namely, leptin and ghrelin, the "yin and yang" of hunger hormones. They work together symbiotically to suppress or stimulate your hunger and satiety in order to maintain weight and energy. Leptin is primarily the satiety hormone; its main objective is to keep the body at a healthy weight, and it lets you know that you've had enough food after a satisfying meal. Produced in specialized cells located in the lining of the stomach and in the pancreas, ghrelin sends hunger cues to the brain when your stomach is empty, prompting you to eat and store fat to then be turned into energy. It also stimulates the reward center in the brain, which is why when we smell, taste, or even think about tasty foods, ghrelin is produced. Think about that great whiff of garlic when you walk into an Italian restaurant or that wonderful mix of turmeric, saffron, and other rich spices in an Indian restaurant.

Because the gut plays such a nuanced role in our appetite, hormone balance, and weight, it's essential to maintain a healthy gut microbiome. The microbiome isn't static; you aren't born with certain gut bacteria and then die with those same microbes. The microbiome is a living organism that changes based on what you eat and other lifestyle factors. We'll get into this much more in chapter

5, but the simple takeaway here is that if we don't take care of our gut diversity, we are affecting much more than how we process our food: you are going to feel so effing tired if your gut microbiome is a mess.

THE BRAIN

While much of the mechanics of the brain remains a mystery, one thing is true: contrary to popular lore, we humans use much more than 10 percent of our brain (we use that much in our sleep). Needless to say, the brain is doing a whole lot of work 24/7, making thousands of decisions in a second, and we now know that the brain controls and communicates with hormones in more ways than we previously suspected. The exact way this is done is not yet clear, but it is key to understanding the brain-hormone connection (more commonly known as the mind-body connection). This is why stress can up your cortisol levels and breathing exercises can tell the brain to relax and lower those levels. Don't believe me? Try this exercise: Breathe in for six counts and exhale for six. Do this three times. Do you notice your breathing is slower? You just lowered your stress hormones!

We are just discovering how all this communication takes place and how to better access this brain-hormone connection, but while there's much to discover, there's a lot we already know about how consistent, chronic stress (or, more technically, sympathetic nervous system activation and the inability to counteract that activation) can cause brain fog and/or low mood, fatigue, lack of concentration, and hormonal imbalances through GnRH pulse disruption. This connection plays a pivotal role in my plan and was key in helping patients like Sherri — and perhaps it will help you too.

HOW TO DETECT
HORMONAL IMBALANCE

Previously I discussed several key hormones that, if unbalanced, can cause the whole hormonal system to falter, zapping your energy and making you feel wiped out. And unfortunately, women are much more vulnerable to hormone imbalance than men, and the likelihood of this imbalance increases with age (oh joy!). No matter what you may have heard about some new test or magical theory, there is no reliable and accurate testing for hormone levels that everyone can agree on. Throughout my extensive work in this area and continued discussions with colleagues, it's just something that remains very controversial. The problem is that hormones are always fluctuating, and their functions are so intertwined that it's hard to capture the big picture. It's important to listen to your body, and if something feels wrong, consult your doctor. Here are some questions you can ask yourself if you think you may have a hormone imbalance.

QUIZ: ARE YOUR HORMONES IN HARMONY?

- Do you feel tired all the time?
- Do you have trouble sleeping?
- Do you feel tired all day but then feel wired at night?
- Do you have frequent mood swings?
- Do you suffer from increased fat storage, especially around the stomach area or the upper thigh area?
- Do you experience frequent headaches, especially new or worsened migraines?
- Do you have increased cravings, either for salty foods, fatty foods, or sugary foods?
- Do you have hives or unexplained rashes?
- For women: Do you have heightened PMS symptoms?
- For men: Do you have lower libido or increased fat storage?

If you answered yes to one or more of these questions, you may have a hormonal imbalance. If you suspect that you have an imbalance, I suggest you see your practitioner and get a full hormone workup and blood work — and, of course, continue reading this book. (See the appendix on page 296 for a list of common diagnostic tests.)

While these tests can be helpful for specific and big, obvious imbalances and perhaps more serious conditions, remember, it is hard to untangle the true underlying cause of hormonal imbalance since having just one hormone out of balance can cause a cascade of inefficiencies in other hormones. It's the combination of these hormones, the collective imbalance, that makes you so effing fatigued.

More about testing: As a society, we put a lot of weight on testing. When things come out negative, relief abounds. The hormonal balance is so complex that it doesn't always show up on tests, so you still may have symptoms even while your blood work and other test results look fine. So I look at testing as just one piece of data. Really, it's a matter of listening to your body and seeing if your symptoms are getting better. That's why if you're tired, anxious, and stressed, there are other diagnostics than tests that are better indicators of what ails you. So, for example, one of the biggest ways to check if you're doing okay (or not) in the microbiome is to check on your energy levels. As technology advances, we should one day be able to use testing to detect imbalances, but for now, early symptoms are best detected by questioning.

We can look for clues from our own bodies. Hormones should work for you instead of against you, and when that hormone system is out of whack, you can work with your doctor to determine if your symptoms point to a hormonal imbalance. It can be a bit of a guessing game, but my plan works on multiple levels that can help rebalance a multitude of hormonal issues.

Take Mary, a lawyer and mother of two, who got breast cancer at the young age of 38. But she got through it — with both surgery and chemo — and licked the disease. She was happy to be free and clear, but after a year she was still feeling really tired. Everyone kept reassuring her that she was clear of cancer and her blood work was "normal." So why did she feel off? More than feeling off, she felt tired all the time. And to make matters worse, at night she would feel "tired and wired."

Frustrated, she came to me for advice. I first reviewed all her history and blood work and then did an exam. I asked her to do some functional exercises like the "sit to stand" exercise, in which you get up from a cross-legged position on the floor without using your hands. (Try it — it is much harder than it looks!) It's a great predictor of longevity.

After talking to her at length — in addition to feeling tired, she had brain fog, weight gain, and sleep issues — it was clear to me that her hormonal axis was off. She had far too much cortisol, which was most likely causing the "traffic jam" and a multitude of symptoms. In her case, both the cancer and its treatment had caused hormonal flux, but as a 40-year-old woman, she was also going through some natural changes that would affect her hormone levels (a part of life every woman looks forward to, right? Ha!). We decided to put her on my plan. After six weeks, she came back, happy to report her progress. "I can't believe it, I feel like I am in a better mood, I am digesting my food better, and most importantly I have *so* much more energy!"

With Mary, we can see that big and small imbalances can put our whole system out of sorts, causing fatigue, zapping your energy, and making you feel stressed, foggy, and run-down. The good news is, just as my plan helped Mary, hormones can be balanced naturally to help regain energy levels.

In the next chapter, we'll discuss *how* exactly we have driven our hormones to distraction and detail how a multitude of lifestyle habits and environmental factors play a role in these hormonal imbalances, including chronic or extreme stress, poor diet, and nutrition. Ready to find out how we effed up our hormones — and how to regain your energy for good?

2

How Did Our Hormones
Get So Effed Up?

SYLVIA WAS IN A PANIC.

"I'm tired, but I can't sleep. I'll fall asleep for a little bit, but then I am up for hours. I'll fall asleep again eventually, only to have to get up an hour later for work," she shared with me, obviously distressed, over our virtual appointment via Zoom. It probably didn't help that Covid was still very much a stressor for everyone. "I am bloated and constipated, and I can feel my pants getting tighter and tighter. But I work out every. Damn. Day. I have insane cravings for sugar in the afternoon, and my PMS is out of control. What is up with me?!"

I told her that I had felt that same frustration. "I remember feeling so out of control as well, because my body was failing me and I could not get a handle on my symptoms, which seemed so unrelated. But they are related, Sylvia. Like you, nothing in all my tests seemed to point to a problem, yet no one could tell me what was wrong with me. But everything my body was telling me was that I was not okay. Is this how you feel?"

"YES!" she let out, with a sigh of relief.

I mentioned all the research that I had done that pointed to my hormones being off-kilter. I had a hunch that she, too, had a myriad of hormone imbalances, something that Western medicine just doesn't have an answer for . . . yet. And the predominant hormone imbalance she seemed to suffer from — cortisol — is one of the most common I see in women.

As we discussed in the first chapter, all our hormones are interconnected, and the smallest imbalance of this axis can present as a myriad of symptoms. For example, just from Sylvia describing her day, I could tell that her cortisol levels were high, and that her melatonin and insulin levels were off. She spent most of her day putting out fires at her job, facing one stressor after another. She was doing intense home cardio workouts after work, and then eating around 9 p.m., which was the earliest she could sit down to a meal given her busy work and exercise schedule.

Here's how Sylvia's day translated to her hormones: The multiple stressful events at work would make her tired during the day, but wired at night. Her workouts added even more stress to her body. Because of this, her sleep suffered. She went to bed late, which delayed her melatonin release, and she went to bed on a full stomach. Eating late at night caused an abnormal insulin spike (because at night our insulin resistance is higher, which gives off a signal to store fat), and it was disrupting her sleep pattern. She would wake up with a spike of cortisol sometimes in the middle of the night between 3 and 5 a.m. Then she'd have a crash in her cortisol levels between 2 and 4 in the afternoon, causing her to have profound fatigue. Desperate to stay alert at work, she would then have something sugary to keep her awake. It was a vicious circle.

Maybe you see yourself in Sylvia. Working long hours, with fitful sleep and food cravings galore. These seemingly disparate symptoms are hard to diagnose, but many crazy hard-to-diagnose symptoms can be linked to our hormones. *How* exactly have we driven our hormones to distraction? Well, as complicated as hormones are, the reasons they get effed up are just as complicated. Even the smallest imbalance can cause major disruptions in different parts of the body; the symptoms can be wide-ranging and the causes difficult to pinpoint. And the way that conventional medicine treats hormone imbalance is complicated. (Because nothing in life is simple, is it?!)

Let's revisit my patient Mary, the 40-year-old cancer survivor. By the time she came to me, she'd had umpteen doctors tell her umpteen different reasons for her fatigue. They assured her that she was fine — they chalked it up to the fact that she was getting older or that she was a busy mom with two kids. She was getting the same brush-offs I heard from my colleagues back when I had my personal energy crisis. Maybe your doctor has said the same things to you. It's not that uncommon these days.

None of what the doctors said was wrong, exactly. Modern medicine is incredible, but there is still so much to learn about hormones and there has yet to be accurate, dependable testing of hormone levels. The tests that do exist to detect hormonal imbalances are only capable of measuring huge disparities, which means they are only good indicators if a hormone is totally out of whack. These tests fail to pick up smaller imbalances that, while perhaps less disruptive than a major imbalance, can greatly affect our energy levels or cause other symptoms that go otherwise underdiagnosed. (Is it any wonder that so many people continue to feel like crap and worry that they are hypochondriacs?)

If Mary had a huge imbalance, her tests would have shown that, but she only had slightly elevated cortisol levels — not enough for tests to pick it up, but certainly enough to give her that draggy, loopy feeling that made her feel off her game. Because her doctors couldn't give her a true diagnosis, she just kept hearing answers like "you're fine" or "you're just getting older." I see a lot of hard-to-detect imbalances like this that are caused by common occurrences, such as menopause, pregnancy, or even PMS, where hormone production may be affected, but not enough to set off alarm bells. So the fatigue continues, untreated.

Let's say Mary's doctors had detected a noticeable decrease in her estrogen levels (instead of her actual issue, which was elevated cortisol). The typical treatment for that is to prescribe natural estrogen or another hormonal product. These natural hormones, in my opinion, have numerous risks, but, more important, the treatment wouldn't have gotten to the root of the problem: what initiated the imbalance in the first place.

Hormones don't just become imbalanced. There has to be a reason that they start going rogue. Our bodies are beautiful intricate machines, and most often it takes something abnormal like an autoimmune disease or cancer to make hormones go off-balance. No one explained this to Mary; no one explained how our hormones work and how they are so essential when it comes to our energy levels. No one told her how, as we discussed in chapter 1, the hormones travel on that interconnected highway that has off-ramps and traffic signals throughout the body, and if there is one slowdown or stoppage, it backs up the entire system.

Now with Mary, perhaps there was a backup on that highway — for some reason her body was making so much cortisol it caused traffic problems, but not enough of a traffic jam to show up on a test. No one informed her that even though the imbalance wasn't off the charts, it could be the cause of her fatigue. It's like saying your car still works, but it's not working very well. It may need new brakes or new tires — you wouldn't want to wait for your car to completely break down to fix it, would you?

When it comes to hormonal imbalance, the source of the problem can be a multitude of lifestyle habits and environmental factors. In this chapter we'll identify the culprits that are effing up our hormones — concentrating on those that have the most to do with our energy levels. As you'll see, many of the causes are rooted in our lifestyle and food choices, our environment, and even our genetics. The good news: while these types of hormonal imbalances may be hard to diagnose, they are easy to fix with lifestyle and dietary changes.

THINGS WE DO TO MESS WITH OUR HORMONES

Over the last hundred years, there has been such a surge in technology and yet a huge decline in our energy levels, which is odd, because you'd think with all the advances that have been made to make our lives easier — cars, cell phones, computers, online retail — that it would be the opposite. It is not an overstatement to say that people suffering from hormonal imbalances have reached epidemic proportions. So what gives? Here are several reasons for this shift.

Stress

You know it, I know it, your next-door neighbor knows it. Chronic stress is not good. We have already talked about how a quick bout of stress can overload your adrenals and increase cortisol — something we'll address more fully in the next chapter — but chronic stress can really be something that may put your overall health at risk in the long run. If your body's stressors are always on, the fight-or-flight reaction that is supposed to be activated for a short period and then go back to baseline also stays on. This can wreak havoc in almost every area of your body and can increase your risk of suffering from a variety of conditions, like anxiety and depression, digestive problems, heart disease, and weight gain. Chronic stress can also destroy the receptors of the hormones — eventually they may stop giving off those bursts of energy, like a lightbulb burning out. Given our modern lifestyle, if we don't take care of ourselves and keep stress under control, it can be a killer.

Our Diet — You Are What You Eat

You've probably heard the phrase "you are what you eat." When it comes to your hormones, this couldn't be more true. For the most part, our hormone glands need cholesterol to produce our hormones, such as cortisol, estrogen, and testosterone. Cholesterol comes from . . . you guessed it, food.

The gut also helps extract food's nutrients in the form of carbohydrates, proteins, and fats that give our body its energy but in different ways. Carbohydrates are best in their fast conversion into sugar to give off quick bursts of energy, and fats are the slowest in delivering energy. When all three are well represented in a diet, carbohydrates and fats are used primarily for energy while protein's main function is to help the body grow, build muscle, and repair. So it is safe to say that what you put in your mouth matters.

Besides knowing the best energy sources that help keep our hormones chugging along, there are a few other key factors that stand out:

Lower food diversity. To me, this is a major disruptor to our hormones. The food we buy today is completely different than the food our grandparents ate even just fifty years ago. Processed foods (i.e., your favorite item at Taco Bell) are filled with salt, sugar, and other bad guys like omega-6 fats and genetically modified ingredients (GMOs). These additives are meant to increase the shelf life of different foods and food products, but they also rip apart our microbiome and mess up our hormones in the process.

What Are GMOs and What Are They Doing in My Food?

While humans have been manipulating plants and animals for thousands of years to yield better-tasting food, recently, due to great strides in technology, there have been more artificial means by which to manipulate the DNA—the genetic code—to garner a better product.

Well, what's wrong with a little innovation? Unfortunately, we don't have enough space in this book to go into all the controversy, but my concern is that we just don't know enough to determine definitively how good or bad genetically modified organisms (GMOs) are for us. While there have been no conclusive studies about the long-term effects of GMO foods on the body, there are theoretical concerns about serious alterations in food's overall compromised nutritional value and the possibilities of toxic effects. Until recently, standards about labeling GMO foods were pretty lax in the United States as opposed to Europe, but in 2016 the federal government put into law that there must be uniform labeling for genetically engineered products.[1] I say be a smart shopper, read labels, and keep on top of the latest research on genetically engineered products.

Highly processed foods also spike glucose levels — and if we eat this way consistently, well, those levels will remain high, giving our insulin levels quite a roller-coaster ride. In general, we are eating too much processed dairy, gluten, and sugary foods, and we are not eating enough prebiotic fiber and vegetables. (We need prebiotics that encourage the growth of "good bacteria," which in turn modulate our hormone levels — we'll discuss this more in chapter 5.)

Even worse, processed foods trick the mind and hoodwink our hunger signals. Your Sunday brunch pancakes or pizza from your favorite delivery place may be delicious, but they are low in protein, an essential nutrient that keeps our blood sugar levels stable, which in turn helps us get that feeling of fullness by reducing levels of ghrelin (the hormone that tells us to eat).

Alcohol

I know, I know, you don't want to hear it. You want me to say that your glass of wine at night is fine by me. But, unfortunately, booze causes your estrogen levels to rise. Studies have shown that women who drink alcohol have higher estrogen levels than teetotalers. And consistent drinkers have been shown to have increased rates of breast cancer, among other estrogen-dominant-related issues. But don't freak out! Drinking moderately, meaning three drinks a week or so, is a way to enjoy your wine (or tequila!) without wrecking your hormones.

Sugar, sugar, sugar. I'm not the first to talk about the dangers of sugar. The media and health advocates have done a great job of getting the word out about how unhealthy sugar is to the body (with creative campaigns such as "drinking soda is the new smoking"). But we still have a long way to go.

Sugar has been integrated into nearly every processed food, so it's a hard habit to break. But we need to: sugar leads to spikes of insulin, causing that traffic on the highway, which in turn creates a cascade of hormonal imbalances (typically in estrogen, testosterone, and progesterone). Foods high in sugar can also hinder the appetite-suppressing hormone leptin — and that, my friends, is why you want to eat an entire bag of chips or a half-dozen donuts. When you consistently eat foods high in sugar, those insulin levels remain chronically high — that is, until your body builds a tolerance to it, causing insulin resistance.[2] (We will go into how to help ourselves get off so much sugar later in the WTF plan.)

Conventional foods. Even when you're avoiding processed foods and eating whole foods, our modern farming practices are working against you. Non-organic dairy, veggies, meat, and fish are filled with their own various levels of hormones. Think about it. Growth hormones are used on commercially raised animals to make them bigger and to increase milk production in cows. These hormones make their way into our food and drink, where they mess with our own hormones.

This is why it's so important to choose organic milk and cheeses that come from cows free of growth hormones, and to avoid veggies laced with pesticides. Nix farm-raised fish that have been fed a high-fat diet and may contain polychlorinated biphenyl, more commonly known as PCB, and other toxins. PCB is a mixture of chemicals that had been used in coolants and lubricants in the past but is no longer produced in the United States, as it has been shown to cause negative health effects, like skin rashes, liver damage, and even cancer in animals. Unfortunately, PCBs can still be found in the environment, typically in bodies of water.[3] Another chemical to watch out for is glyphosate — an herbicide widely used on crops and plants

(Roundup is the most famous brand). It can be found on produce, in meat, packaged foods (such as Ritz Crackers and Oreos!), even in water. While studies conflict, there is an increasing body of research showing that glyphosate is a hormone disruptor that can lead to a multitude of issues like reproductive problems, cancer, and diabetes.[4] It can also affect our sacred gut bacteria. While the FDA currently has no regulation against it, the World Health Organization has called it a "probable carcinogen." So I would stay away. Who wants that crap in your body?

IT'S ALL ABOUT TIMING

We are our own worst enemy. I'll say it again: Our bodies were made to be nearly perfect running machines. The body runs like clockwork—literally—to give you enough energy to get you through the day, and it continues to work at night as you sleep. When we stay up late, eat at odd hours, and deal with chronic stress, we upset this natural circadian rhythm, your body's 24-hour biological cycle that exists in every cell in your body. The body needs to rest so it is able to repair itself. Those actions cannot happen when you are always trying to metabolize food or when you're in a state of stress. Alterations of circadian biology due to modern life—too much exposure to the blue lights of our cell phones, city living, traveling to different time zones, eating late—have a largely disruptive effect on our cells and hormone production. (We'll get more into all of this in chapter 6.)

And this is why it is as important to talk about *when* to eat as much as it is about what you eat. You may have heard about intermittent fasting (IF)—eating in a restricted window of time, usually 8–12 hours in any given day. Typically people who try intermittent fasting opt to eat in an 8-hour window such as 12 p.m. to 8 p.m., so they are essentially skipping breakfast but still eating their last meal somewhat late at night.

While this may follow the typical IF rules, it's actually not working with your body for maximum results, especially if you (like most of us) make dinner your heaviest meal of the day. There is a more specific way of fasting that I suggest to my patients: fasting in tune with your own circadian rhythm. Time-restricted eating within certain hours has been shown to trigger such good effects as decreased inflammation and improved metabolic function. This may have to do with melatonin — the hormone that helps us sleep.

Groundbreaking research on circadian rhythm by the Salk Institute's Dr. Satchin Panda — a worldwide leader in circadian rhythm studies and the author of *The Circadian Code: Lose Weight, Supercharge Your Energy, and Sleep Well Every Night* — shows that when our bodies are working optimally, melatonin will start to kick in 2–3 hours after we last eat; it also signals to the pancreas to stop producing insulin. If you eat a meal late in the day, your pancreas cannot handle the load since melatonin has already told it to shut down for the night. Your body thought it was supposed to be resting and repairing, but all of a sudden it has to digest food. This can affect our health in many ways, including causing a dysfunctional insulin response and triggering metabolic syndrome — and, you guessed it, weight gain. Studies have also shown that elevated blood sugar levels may affect brain health, memory, and cognition. Worse, it doesn't take a lot to increase that insulin and hinder your melatonin — even a relaxing late-night glass of sauvignon blanc can be bad for you.

If you're always eating or sleeping at a time that doesn't align with your internal clock, you are going to be activating pathways that shouldn't be activated. If that highway is filled with cars instead of leaving the roads open so your hormones can do the nightly roadwork needed to restore and repair your systems, you're going to get an inevitable traffic jam, and that much-needed repair won't get done. And your hormones aren't going to like it. That's why resetting and restoring this natural circadian rhythm to keep your hormones happy is a big part of my plan. I combine the ideals of intermittent fasting while keeping in mind the importance of our circadian rhythm, so your last bite will be well before you hit the hay. (So instead of an eating window of 12 p.m. to 8 p.m., I'll be recommending a window of 9 a.m. to 6 p.m.) But more on that later.

OUR ENVIRONMENT

Today we live in a world that is filled with so many chemicals and genetically modified foods that it can throw our system completely out of balance, especially our hormones. Think about it. After a workout —one of the healthiest things you can do—right away you probably reach for water . . . in a plastic bottle. Depending on the bottle, the plastic could contain parabens and other chemicals, particularly BPA, a chemical found in several plastics and plastic additives that can mimic the hormone estrogen. The industry has caught on to this, and while we have seen a flood of new BPA-free plastic products, a new study shows that even if plastic products don't contain BPA, most still release chemicals that are similar to estrogen.[5] In this study, a plastic product (e.g., a baby bottle) can consist of a hundred or more chemicals (including pesticides, as well as parabens that also mimic estrogen). Beyond being gross, this is really bad for our health —those chemicals can leach from the plastic product into our food and water![6] Look around your kitchen and bathroom, and you'll find a shocking number of products with chemicals that can wreak havoc with your hormones: bottles, plastic wrap, plastic food containers, beauty products, medications, makeup. I could go on (in fact, I did —see the box on page 67). Think about all the products that touch your food and your body *every day*. This impostor estrogen from environmental chemicals is like a stolen car on the highway—it is going to mess with that traffic flow and create imbalances throughout the body.

Ticktock: Perimenopause and Menopause

Perimenopause usually begins several years before menopause kicks in, starting in our forties. During this time, our ovaries start to produce less and less estrogen. When our bodies finally put the brakes on releasing eggs altogether, well, I can almost hear Oprah singing, "Welcome to *MENOPAAUUUUSE!*" You might as well sign up for AARP membership benefits and half-priced senior movie tickets, right? Nah. While for many years doctors prescribed hormone replacement therapy (HRT) to alleviate symptoms of menopause (like hot flashes, low libido, weight gain, loss of muscle composition, mood swings), there are many ways to ameliorate these symptoms and make up for the body's loss of estrogen naturally.

HRT remains the proverbial elephant in the room, as the controversial treatment has gone in and out of favor for years. (Just like fashion, as Heidi Klum says, "One day you're in; the next day you're out.") My opinion is to take HRT seriously and talk to your doctor. He or she can run some tests and determine what is right for you; with my patients, I first have them try lifestyle and diet changes, and what I have found is that 90 percent never need exogenous hormones. For the small minority who do need HRT, it has to be done with very thoughtful consideration that weighs the risks with benefits.

My patient Michelle, an interior designer in her thirties, was struggling with weight loss. She did all the tried-and-true things that helped her lose weight before, but they didn't seem to be working anymore. She was still gaining weight, especially in her thighs (oy). She also noticed that her premenstrual syndrome (PMS) symptoms were much more pronounced, and so she wondered if her issues were hormone related.

I asked her questions related to other hormonal symptoms and suspected she likely was suffering from estrogen dominance, which is very common in the US because as women we use products that contain estrogen-like compounds every day (like makeup). Pile on the fun fact that Michelle was getting older, so getting rid of all this excess estrogen gets extra hard. And it's not about adding progesterone to balance out the higher estrogen levels; we needed to really bring the estrogen levels down.

So I told Michelle to clean out her bathroom cabinets to get rid of any BPA or paraben-filled personal care products. I also suggested that she add cruciferous veggies like broccoli and rocket to her diet — these kinds of veggies have the naturally occurring compound indole-3-carbinol, which works to balance estrogen. I also asked her to try to reduce her cortisol by doing breathing exercises: 15 minutes in the morning to get ready for the day and 15 minutes at night to decompress.

Guess what? In three months, she was markedly better.

Xenoestrogens

The media and the clean-living movement have helped create tremendous awareness about the harmful products and ingredients that surround us. And there has been much to-do around xenoestrogens — industrial chemicals that mimic the behavior of estrogens. In fact, you may already know a lot about which products to avoid, but it's incredible how many chemicals still surround us in our everyday lives, from our water bottles to hygiene products to our food, so you need to stay vigilant about what you are putting on and into your body. Here's a list of ingredients to watch out for.

BPA: First, BPA (bisphenol A) is a synthetic estrogen used in countless plastic products like water and soda bottles, baby bottles and children's toys, and fast food packaging. Even those carbonless cash register receipts we get from pharmacies, gas stations, and grocery stores contain BPA. The interactions we have with such plastic may seem minor, but even small amounts of exposure can affect us. BPA can be absorbed through the skin, ingested, or inhaled.[7] It can also be found in metal cans used for canned veggies and fruits, where it is used to keep aluminum from leaching into the food. What to do? Well, go back to basics. Eat on real dishes — glass, ceramic, or stainless steel — and use real silverware and skip fast-food burgers altogether.

Parabens: Parabens are also endocrine disruptors, and your medicine cabinet is probably filled with them. These synthetic compounds are frequently used in much of our hair and beauty products like shampoos and conditioners, makeup, and moisturizers. Scarily, they are easily absorbed by the human body. One study found that 99 percent of malignant breast cancer tumors contained one to five different types of parabens.[8] They can also lead to various developmental, hormonal, and neurological disorders. Be on the lookout for any ingredients that end with "paraben" like methylparaben or butylparaben.[9] The good news is that thanks to growing awareness about these chemicals, it's easier to find clean beauty and bathroom products. (For more information, check out EWG.org.)

The bottom line is there is a lot out there waiting to eff us up: the stress in our lives, the way we eat, and what we buy can all have huge effects on our hormone health. Be good to yourself — and the planet. Stay away from plastics, BPAs, and parabens as much as possible, and follow the WTF diet plan to help you on your way to optimizing your hormones (and your energy) instead of impairing them.

Now let's look at another major hormonal imbalance — so-called adrenal fatigue — which is such a behemoth it gets its own chapter.

3

Adrenal Fatigue Is Not Just About the Adrenals

AFTER MY ACCIDENT, I searched for reasons why I was so super tired. Poring over my medical books and journals, but not finding any answers to what the heck was wrong with me, I got a little desperate. So I, like most of you, I'm sure, googled my symptoms. (Yes, even doctors are sometimes guilty of this, even though we officially preach to our patients to do otherwise! I promise, I don't make it a habit.) These are the myriad questions I googled:

- Why am I so fatigued?
- Why do I have insomnia?
- What do sweet and salty cravings mean?
- Am I addicted to caffeine?
- Why am I having constipation and feeling bloated?

I scoured hundreds of websites, blogs, forums, and media pieces looking for my answer. And over and over, I kept reading about a condition with which I was not familiar: "adrenal fatigue," or AF.

It was all over the internet: "Do You Have Adrenal Fatigue?" "Adrenal Fatigue Got You Down?" "What Vitamins Are Good for AF?" Even the "Adrenal Fatigue Diet." In a 2016 study on adrenal fatigue, the authors found that when they searched "adrenal fatigue" on Google, it provided 640,000 results, and the association of the two words exhibited 1.54 million findings.[1]

So how come I had never heard of it? All my symptoms pointed to it, yet in my medical training, with all the studying I had conducted on the adrenal glands and their function (adrenaline, aldosterone, and cortisol production), why had I never heard of adrenal fatigue? I have vivid memories of studying the adrenals in my anatomy lab: I just stared at the tiny organ. It was the weight of four paper clips. *How did something so tiny do so much for our bodies,* I remember thinking.

But I never heard about AF, except in the form of adrenal dysfunction in the very serious condition called Addison's disease, in which the adrenal glands just don't work to full compacity and can't produce enough cortisol. But it is rare, and it can be so serious that a lot of sufferers can become immobile, so I knew that is not what I had. Unfortunately, AF has become a hugely popular catchphrase in the wellness and health ecosystem, so it's hard to know what is true and what isn't.

My internet findings were met with amusement from my colleagues, and my ensuing questions were dismissed. "Never heard of such a thing," my doctor colleagues would say. But I *knew* something was off with my hormones because I was so effing tired all the time. So I did additional research, and I found out that both camps were right. "Adrenal fatigue" does not exist — in a biological sense, anyway — but the symptoms associated with it do. How can this be? Because the hormonal axis is just so darn complicated and intertwined that an imbalance isn't usually just from one source. Think of your hormones like a game of Jenga — when everything is stacked together evenly, the delicate tower can hold. But all it takes is one hormone imbalance to throw the tower out of balance and create a cascade in which other hormones become imbalanced, causing everything to crumble.

Because this interdependent axis is so hard to diagnosis, doctors and practitioners should take their patients seriously when they do exhibit these symptoms and not brush it off as "you're fine, just get some more rest" or "you're just stressed out." The symptoms are there; we just need to diagnose these seemingly disparate symptoms in a broader, more complex way. Patients shouldn't have to resort to Dr. Google to get to the bottom of their persistent fatigue, cravings, and chronic stress. Let's cut out the noise from the ether, and discover the truth about the adrenals, hormonal imbalance, and what you can do to reclaim your energy (and your life!).

IF IT'S NOT AF, WHAT IS IT?

Alternative health proponents of AF talk of "adrenal exhaustion" as the culprit for our batteries going dangerously low. As you read in an earlier chapter, the adrenals are two small glands that rest atop the kidneys and produce several hormones, cortisol being one of them. When you're under stress, short bursts of cortisol get released into the bloodstream. Advocates of AF claim that prolonged exposure to stress could drain the adrenals of cortisol. The adrenal depletion would cause brain fog, low energy, depressive mood, salt and sweet cravings, light-headedness, and other vague symptoms.

Actually the opposite happens. Simply put, when you're stressed, the adrenal glands actually produce *more* cortisol — they don't stop because you are stressed. I know what you are thinking: *Okay, so if AF is really not a diagnosis, that doesn't take away the fact that I still feel like crap. For sure, something is going on.* The symptoms are real, but the diagnosis is not.

What is really happening is a cortisol imbalance.

❧

Maria was in her early thirties with three kids and a demanding career as a financial analyst when she came to me because she felt overly tired. She was first seduced by the AF theory, but then she didn't feel any better after working with an "adrenal fatigue" expert and taking what seemed like a zillion different vitamins. Maria's lab work showed that she had high blood sugar. Even though her other hormone tests came out negative (because, as explained on page 57, only major imbalances will show up in testing), her elevated blood sugar levels were a clue that something was off.

I explained to Maria that her emergency response system was on overdrive, but that this didn't mean she had "adrenal fatigue." I told her about how the adrenals are part of an interconnected hormonal highway, and if one hormonal gland malfunctions, it will impact everything on this highway and your overall health will suffer. So if your thyroid or adrenal glands are functioning at a suboptimal level, it is a systemic issue and not a singular, isolated problem — think about NYC during rush hour, and how a traffic jam on one street can snarl traffic in a larger area. This is why it's crucial to look at your full hormonal picture — and it is precisely why hormonal imbalances are difficult to pinpoint.

So what, exactly, was happening with Maria's hormones? We have talked about the fight-or-flight trigger that is driven by the sympathetic nervous system, a coordinated network of brain receptors, nerves, and hormones that, when working normally, directs your involuntary response to stress: heart rate and breathing go up, eyes dilate, and an infusion of glucose is shot into the bloodstream for a quick energy boost. When the perceived threat is gone, the back end of the nervous system — the parasympathetic nervous system — kicks in to slow everything down. When in harmony, the sympathetic and parasympathetic systems work together to maintain homeostasis.

Maria's problem was that she was staying in that sympathetic mode all the time — her body felt like it was in a constant emergency situation. This affected her body in a myriad of ways: her gut couldn't function properly because she was hardly ever in the parasympathetic "rest and digest" mode, which tells your body it's time to digest and repair. It's the opposite of fight or flight, the mode we are in when we are scared or stressed.

Her hormones were out of whack because of cortisol being stolen from the other hormones, the pregnenolone steal syndrome discussed earlier. In addition, her immune system was malfunctioning due to the miscommunication between gut bacteria and immune cells.

This "stuck" mode is prevalent with busy women. I have another patient, Malika, a former college athlete who is now a working mom in her thirties without any free time for exercise. She's leading a sedentary life, and her diet, well, what diet? She skips meals, but snacks on the kids' leftover snacks. Her work life is busy, with urgent emails that keep her in sympathetic mode. Tina, another athlete patient of mine, was in her twenties and still worked out (hard) every day. But in the midafternoon, she'd crash and would "need" two or three cups of coffee to get her through the rest of the day. The fuel for her intense workouts was limited — and she often drove up her cortisol and adrenaline levels (which were already high from lack of sleep and stress) by exercising. This constant sympathetic hormone surge leads to high blood sugar and possibly pregnenolone steal (see page 39). (We still don't know if this latter process actually exists, but it is a popular theory among functional-health professionals.) What we do know is that all of these women have a sympathetic system on overdrive — not AF.

The good news is that even though this is common, there is hope. I had Maria (like other patients) do the two-week WTF plan, and she saw a vast improvement: she had more even energy, a better mood, and decreased blood sugar.

Please Don't Take Supplements for AF

As you probably already know, the FDA does not regulate the supplement industry, a multibillion-dollar business that's based on selling you products that you think you want or need to stay healthy. Unfortunately, without FDA oversight, no one can really say how effective these supplements are, or how much is actually safe to take. I have many patients come to me after taking so-called adrenal hormone supplements

that are meant to support adrenal function. The trouble
with this is that these supplements aren't known to be
effective (remember: AF isn't an actual disease, according
to the Endocrine Society), and they could cause more harm
than good.

How? If you take supplements unnecessarily, your adrenal
glands may become unable to produce the hormones when
you really do need them. Worse, taking supplements like this
creates an increased risk of developing the life-threatening
condition of adrenal crisis.[2]

While Maria, Tina, and Malika were in their twenties and thirties, many women in their forties, fifties, and beyond are also affected by sympathetic system overdrive. One of my patients, Donna, who was perimenopausal, was doing everything right — eating healthfully and exercising regularly — but her periods were exaggerated and she was having trouble sleeping because of stress about her aging parents (hello, Facebook friends, who else is up at 4 a.m.?). Her periods seemed to last *forever*, and she developed weird food sensitivities that caused bloating, constipation, and also sleep issues. To best describe what is going on with Donna's hormones, picture a nearly empty tube of toothpaste. Squeezing that tube, sometimes you get a great smooth paste, but sometimes it sputters or too much comes out all at once. Irregularities happen when this sympathetic mode begets pregnenolone steal.

. . . AND MODERN LIFE IS TO BLAME

So why is sympathetic overload so common? We bombard our very sensitive system with daily stresses — think family, work, the 24/7 news cycle, and social media. Not to mention the fact that we've virtually forgotten how to relax, play, and take a moment for ourselves. I could go on and on.

A few years ago, on a trip to visit family in India, I remember marveling how people in all the different small towns we visited had the same wonderful idea: they'd meet up on their stoops at teatime and chat for hours with their neighbors. They'd allowed themselves to take time after dinner to walk, socialize, and connect with people, which, studies have shown, is so vital to our overall well-being. No one was eating in a car, honking at the stopped traffic, chugging their Starbucks coffee as they hustled down the street, or still at the office at 9 p.m. All around the world, outside of the US, communities understand the importance of personal downtime and connection. Fatigue and hormonal problems seem to be at nearly epidemic proportions across this country — bound by our very own self-imposed, competitive, rushed, and hectic lives. I don't have accurate statistics, but I would say sympathetic overload isn't such a problem elsewhere in the world because of the value other cultures place on work-life balance and daily self-care. A recent study showed that most people in Europe (France, Germany, Spain, and the United Kingdom) logged more than 30 days of vacation and holidays, while those in the US only logged 10 days.[3] With that kind of time off, we can only imagine how much stress levels differ across the pond.

Adrenal Insufficiency

While AF is something of an alternative health urban myth, don't confuse AF with adrenal insufficiency, a true medical condition where the adrenals fail to produce cortisol. Also known as Addison's disease, the relatively rare disease is usually caused by an autoimmune issue, and its symptoms usually come on slowly. In addition to weight loss, its symptoms include joint pain, vomiting, and diarrhea. Unlike other hormonal imbalances, there is actually a pretty accurate test for diagnosing it.[4]

WHAT TO DO ABOUT IT

Here's the thing about cortisol imbalance. Not only is it a problem in and of itself, but it's also the main driver of other hormonal imbalances. So improving your cortisol levels and balancing your adrenaline levels are going to help any other hormone problem you might have.

Part of the issue with cortisol imbalance is that your adrenal organs are getting immune to high levels of cortisol. And so you are producing a ton of cortisol, which, if you remember from chapter 2, is not easy for your body to produce and takes away precursors from other hormones. On top of that, you are getting a lowered response every time you produce it. Cortisol is continuously being produced, along with adrenaline.

This means that most people with cortisol imbalance will benefit from doing techniques to lower their cortisol and take a break from this constant bombardment of cortisol and adrenaline. This is what I recommend for patients like Maria, Donna, and Tina. We need to turn off cortisol production in the sympathetic nervous system and turn on the opposite system, the parasympathetic nervous system. This "rest and digest" system helps you retain energy by slowing down your heart rate and intestinal tract.

As we strive to balance the parasympathetic system with the sympathetic system, this doesn't mean that it's going to be one-to-one. You're not going to be in parasympathetic mode in equal time. You just need bits of parasympathetic mode during the day. One of my favorite ways to turn on this parasympathetic mode is vagal stimulation, which is the main nerve responsible for turning on the parasympathetic response. Something as simple as deep breathing exercises can easily stimulate the vagal nerve. Try this exercise: take three long breaths — six counts in and six counts out. Feel the difference? These slow, deep breaths actually stimulate the big old nervous system — the vagal nerve — to turn on. That's why yoga and meditation is so effective for managing cortisol levels: it automatically makes you slow down your breathing and activate that vagal nerve, which then turns on the parasympathetic response that has such healing properties in our bodies.

This parasympathetic nervous system not only relaxes your body and turns off the sympathetic system, it also turns on the digestive processes and the repair processes. Remember how I said in chapter 1 that the gut and hormones are closely related? You can imagine how someone who is constantly in sympathetic mode is going to have GI troubles because their food is not allowed to digest. If you're constantly in that fight-or-flight mode, you're not allowing yourself to digest properly because your body is concentrating on sending blood flow to the main muscles (in preparation for a perceived fight or flight) instead. Your brain function and repair functions also suffer.

Stimulating the vagal nerve with deep breathing is perhaps one of the easiest techniques for bringing your hormones back into balance. But it's not the only one. (I'll go into greater detail about this plan later in the book.)

᳞

Adrenal fatigue may be the "it girl" of medical conditions on popular health and wellness sites and books, but don't believe the hype. And always work with your doctor before getting sucked into any products, supplements, or programs you read about online. Getting a definitive diagnosis is really what you need, because otherwise you may be wasting your time when you actually have something serious going on. Your health is too important, and your symptoms may be a sign of other conditions, like anemia, autoimmune diseases, infections, other hormonal imbalances, or heart and lung problems. Get tested to look into the true cause of your fatigue, and of course look into lifestyle changes (that much-needed sleep, getting more fiber in your diet, reducing your stress — you know the drill) that can improve your hormone system overall — and your energy levels.

Next, we'll look at another key issue — inflammation — that can seriously mess with your energy.

4

Inflammation Is an Energy Leech

A COUPLE OF YEARS AGO, I bought a new pair of killer heels for a business trip to New York City. My feet looked great in the chic red-soled pumps as I walked down Fifth Avenue like I owned it. (When you are barely five feet tall, not only are heels a great fashion statement, but they are also your best accessory.) I was rocking it until the smallest crack in the sidewalk caused me to lose my balance. My ankle went one way as the rest of my leg went the other way, and I fell hard onto the cold, harsh reality of Manhattan pavement. My ankle swelled up like a balloon and felt warm to the touch. It hurt like a mofo, but I wasn't worried. I took a minimal amount of ibuprofen because I knew that the pain and swelling were indicators that my immune system was working and I was healing. After all my years in the medical profession, I still find the body's natural healing response incredible. I let my body do its thing, giving my ankle as much rest and elevation as possible, and within a few weeks I was back in heels, opting for fashion over safety (do we ever learn?).

Think about the last time you twisted your ankle, cut your finger, or caught a cold that gave you a sore, swollen throat. Pain and swelling are telltale signs that your body's own defense system is at work. Described by the ancient Greeks as "the internal fire," our protective immune system takes on incoming threats, big and small — like injury, infection, or even foods that our body doesn't recognize. The immune response reacts by increasing blood flow to the affected area, along with a surge of infection-fighting white blood cells and substances called cytokines to fight off infection or other foreign organisms and to help with tissue repair. The result? The area swells up, gets inflamed, and you will feel pain and sometimes have a temporary loss of function, but that inflammation is a good thing. Your immune system kicks in and your cut will eventually heal, your ankle will get better, and your sore throat eventually goes away (with the help of lots of rest, hot tea and lemon, and Netflix). Inflammation is a surefire sign that your immune system is working as it should.

THE FLIP SIDE OF INFLAMMATION

But inflammation is a tricky thing. And when it comes to inflammation, we want just the right amount — we don't want too little or too much of it.

Acute inflammation is a normal response to injury, but it is meant to be temporary. This acute inflammation is good — your body responds to emergencies and then the inflammation recedes after the immune system has done its job. But when too many pro-inflammatory catalysts have built up in us (by lack of sleep, stress, or a poor diet), that inflammatory response gets stuck on high gear and remains high, or chronic.

That's when our immune system goes from doing good to doing harm. Your emergency response system doesn't turn off, consistently trying to put out fires — whether in the form of something you ate that's triggering an immune response or chronic stress — and it never gets a break. It gets confused with the constant bombardment of these modern assaults and starts an autoimmune reaction, which is when the body attacks its own cells by mistake. At that point, the immune system becomes weaker and the body becomes more susceptible to infections and disease. And what is scarier is that we often don't even know it is happening.

When I learned about the fact that the immune system has the power to do both — create inflammation for good and create inflammation that causes disease — it was eye-opening. This dichotomy is a key point when it comes to the energy trifecta. If the immune system spends too much time on high alert, it sucks up all our energy. All of our energy is going to fight off perceived offenders and dangers rather than helping fuel normal body functioning. The immune system also creates cytokines — molecules that are released to the tissue as an immune response. This secretion adds to the feeling of low energy when our bodies have been compromised, say with the flu. When we remain in that high-alert response system too long, we can get a cascade of issues and usher in a string of long-term effects, such as disease and chronic conditions. And its number one symptom: fatigue.

Simply put, chronic inflammation is an energy leech.

The Energy Trifecta

You may already have read a lot about inflammation by now — it has been a health buzzword for several years, and many books, diets, and programs center around reducing chronic inflammation for good reason: it can be so detrimental to our bodies, both in the short term and the long term. Here's the thing: Chronic inflammation is the developed world's silent killer. In 2014 nearly 60 percent of Americans had at least one chronic condition, 42 percent had more than one, and 12 percent of adults had five or more chronic conditions. Worldwide, three out of five people die due to chronic inflammatory diseases like stroke, chronic respiratory diseases, heart disorders, cancer, obesity, and diabetes.[1]

So one peg of that energy trifecta is about keeping inflammation in check to unlock our energy resources. Like the three bears' porridge, where Goldilocks wanted it not too hot or too cold, you don't want your inflammatory response to be too little or too long. You want it *just right*. We need to keep it in balance — we need enough to keep us safe from viruses and toxins, as well as to heal wounds. But we don't want too much, where we have *chronic* low-level inflammation, because this can set off a cascade of problems that mess with our hormones, wreak havoc on our gut, and can be the root cause of more serious diseases like diabetes, heart disease, obesity, hypertension, cancer, depression, and anxiety. If not balanced and nurtured, the energy trifecta can all too easily become a sickness trifecta. And since inflammation can be "silent" or difficult to detect, it may be eating away at your quality of life right now, leaving you feeling rundown, blue, or achy, and you don't even know why.

So you might be wondering: Do you have inflammation in your body right now? The answer is an unequivocal yes. A better question to ask is: Do you have inflammation that's chronic and low level, that is causing harm to your blood vessels, your muscles, and your hormone balance? If you have symptoms like headaches, bloating, joint pain, rashes, weight gain, allergies, asthma, or mood issues — you are most likely inflamed.

Autoimmune Diseases

Asthma, allergies, and other autoimmune disorders like celiac disease and rheumatoid arthritis are inflammatory-based diseases that can be triggered when your energy trifecta is off. For reasons unknown, cases of autoimmune diseases in the United States are rising every year, based on a 2020 survey conducted by the National Institute of Environmental Health Sciences, which is part of the NIH.[2] In another survey, the rate of asthma cases is increasing every year: the Centers for Disease Control and Prevention (CDC) reported that between the years of 2001 and 2011, the incidence of asthma increased by 25 percent; the highest increase was among Black children (with a 50 percent increase) from 2001 to 2009.[3] While scientists continue to try to figure out why this is happening, it's more important than ever to cut out inflammatory foods.

Most of you may not even realize you have this inflammation, but you may notice your energy is null and void. Zippo. Your immune system is so busy dealing with all the crap that we eat and do — so many insults on a daily basis — that it's always in reactive mode, and all your energy is so busy covering your immune system that it has time for little else.

And thus it makes us tired. In the long run, when the immune system is in overdrive and this becomes chronic, it triggers a wide range of symptoms from daily headaches and bloating to more serious conditions like Alzheimer's, heart disease, and even certain cancers. Inflammation also allows plaque to accumulate in arteries, leading to heart disease, and is associated with depression, anxiety, and other mood disorders. You're likely getting the message by now — getting your inflammation under control is vital for you to regain your energy and optimize your health.

We want our immune system to be armed and ready to heal our bodies from an injury like a cut, but we don't want it working on overload and causing chronic inflammation. And our over-exercising, overeating, over-stimulated lifestyles cause exactly that. This chronic inflammation is also the real reason you get symptoms of "aging" like aches, pains, and the almighty fatigue.

Signs of Silent Inflammation

Without rigorous testing, it's hard to pinpoint where inflammation is coming from, but there are some signs you may be inflamed:

- Persistent joint or muscle pain
- Constant fatigue or lethargy
- Skin problems
- Inability to lose weight

- Bloating
- Brain fog, focus/memory issues
- PMS (for women)
- Moody, depressed, irritated, frustrated, angry
- Sleeplessness
- Food sensitivities
- Allergies, asthma, eczema
- High blood-glucose levels; high blood pressure
- Diagnosis of diabetes, heart disease, cancer, Alzheimer's, ulcers, IBS, or another inflammatory condition

Top causes of inflammation:

- Stress (physical, emotional, mental)
- Lack of sleep
- Diet high in sugar, carbs, and processed foods
- Diet high in trans fats
- Diet high in omega-6 fatty acids/low in omega-3 fatty acids
- Food allergies or sensitivities
- Alcohol/drug use
- Working out too hard
- Environmental toxins including heavy metals, pesticides, and pollution
- Acute, chronic illness (obesity, lupus, Crohn's)

My patient Sally is a perfect example of someone who was experiencing many of the classic symptoms of chronic inflammation. A busy corporate lawyer and mom of two, the 41-year-old is always on the go. She barely had time to make meals for herself, let alone keep up with her legal briefs, so she ate a lot of processed and sugary foods as she worked. At night, she liked to have a cocktail (or two) to unwind.

Sally came to me because she was experiencing a vague set of symptoms: fatigue, weight gain, and anxiety. I ran some tests, including a thyroid panel, diabetes test, and inflammatory markers, such as the hs-CRP test (see list of possible tests on page 296). Some markers on those tests came back positive, and so I wasn't surprised to find that she was inflamed, meaning her immune system — a key part of the energy trifecta — was out of balance. And because the energy trifecta is so intertwined, when you have one imbalance, it creates an overall imbalance. In Sally's case, because of chronic inflammation, her body reacted with a hormonal imbalance: she released too much of that almighty cortisol too often, causing hormone disruption throughout the body, which in turn affected her gut health. But by healing her chronic inflammation, we were able to bring her entire system back into balance, so that she could feel better and have more energy to fuel her busy days. (We'll get into more detail about how these three systems are interrelated in chapter 7.)

Being Fatigued Can Lead to ... More Fatigue

Our immune system and energy levels are intertwined in a way most people don't understand, but the medical community continues to learn more and more about how they work. A study showed that inflammation in a particular part of the body (for the study, the inflammation was in the liver) can inflame tissue and blood vessels in the brain. This in turn makes our brain perform sub-optimally and creates a feeling of fatigue and can lead to anxiety and even depression. Historically, we thought that the brain was immune to inflammation happening elsewhere in the body, but this promising study shows that the brain is ground zero of our defense system, as it can sense inflammation happening in other parts of the body.[4] Whether it's from a poor diet or lack of sleep, your body will struggle working overtime to put out "fires" throughout your body. The body is designed to go into triage mode when it registers inflammation: it will focus its energy on the inflamed area, all the while depleting resources and energy in other areas.

Everyone is different and has a unique response to different triggers. Still, for many people, certain foods can be a major culprit in inflammation. If you think about it, this makes total sense: food is exogenous, meaning it comes from outside the body. It's only natural that our bodies will flag foods that seem foreign to it, including foods that weren't readily available to our human ancestors, like processed foods — think Doritos and lunchmeat — and our body reacts to it negatively, which causes inflammation. Foods like dairy, gluten (a protein found in wheat and wheat products), alcohol, sugar, and omega-6 oils all cause inflammation.

The good news is that while it is hard to diagnostically test which foods cause inflammation in the body, with some targeted tweaks and adjustments to your lifestyle, you can reduce inflammation quite drastically. And alleviating chronic inflammation is what doctors and big pharma are finding is the "secret" to aging and longevity. The idea behind it is pretty simple: if we can keep inflammation at bay, we can keep a lot of disease that ages us at bay. While traditional medicine continues to focus on fighting inflammation with drugs, studies have shown a direct link between diet and inflammation and illness, as well as how the right foods can help battle and fend off inflammation, giving you the energy you need and keeping you healthier longer.

Take Ella, for example, a 46-year-old real estate attorney who has rheumatoid arthritis. She was used to dealing with inflammation in her joints every day, but then she noticed she had been getting very tired. On top of that, her periods were irregular and very painful, and she complained of weight gain and brain fog. All these signs pointed to a hormone imbalance. And it was affecting her life, so much so that she had to stop teaching art classes at the local community college. She tried traditional treatment — ibuprofen and an immunosuppressive medication — which helped with the pain but not with the fatigue. I coached Ella through my program, and we lowered her sugar intake (she loved her chocolate) and upped her good fatty acids — and her inflammation symptoms disappeared. Her fatigue improved so much she was able to resume teaching the art classes she loved so much.

... and Weight Gain

Jennifer, another patient of mine, at 33 was gaining weight despite a crazy exercise regimen. Her fatigue wouldn't let up, and she noticed that she looked — and felt — older than she should. Inflammation plays a significant role in metabolic syndrome and weight gain. There are a few mechanisms that cause insulin resistance, which in turn leads to making the number on your scale go up and up. New research shows that weight gain in and of itself can become fuel for the inflammatory fire, making it not just harder to lose weight, but causing additional weight gain. That's because fat cells contribute to chronic inflammation, and weight gain, especially in the form of fat tissue, also contributes to chronic inflammation.

How does this work? As we gain weight, some fat cells are forced to expand beyond their typical capacity while trying to store our extra calories as fat. When this happens, they turn on and *add* to the inflammation already present in our bodies. At this point, these cells aren't just fat storage warehouses — they're like little inflammation factories, sending out signals to activate the immune system. Losing weight allows the fat cells to shrink back to a more normal size and turns off the signals that trigger chronic inflammation.

There are a few emerging studies that demonstrate this. In a 2008 UK study, researchers followed people over nine years and monitored things like weight gain and blood levels of C-reactive protein (CRP), a chemical that shows up when the immune system is activated.[5] They found something interesting: weight increases were associated with more inflammation, and the relationship was linear. This means that as a person's weight increased, so did the level of CRP in their blood. There are also a few studies that suggest losing weight should help; one 2004 study by Wake Forest University found that inflammation decreased among participants who went on a low-calorie diet to lose weight.[6] Since losing weight helps decrease inflammation, it may also lower our risk for chronic illnesses, although more studies are needed to prove this link. But this much is clear: inflammation can cause weight gain, which causes more fat cells, which induces more inflammation and more insulin resistance. A vicious cycle.

In Jennifer's case, her cortisol levels were way too high because she was exercising so much; we brought down those cortisol and stress levels by not only decreasing the number of her workout sessions but also having her mix it up with restorative exercise like yoga, and she started to feel like a better version of herself. We stopped the cycle of inflammation, and she could feel the pounds coming off her.

Chronic Inflammation Can Be a Sign of a Leaky Gut

Intestinal inflammation creates what we call a leaky gut, which influences not only our digestion, but overall health and neurobiology, and it is a huge source of inflammation elsewhere. We'll get into leaky gut much more in chapter 5, but the term means what it says: your intestines start to become looser and more porous, letting food particles from your gut seep into your bloodstream. Gross, right? Since your immune system constantly guards the gut border, it sees these particles as intruders and attacks them.[7] Typically, an "intruder" — say, the protein from gluten — travels through the gut epithelia, which is the intestine lining that plays a critical role in preventing anything from getting past that layer.[8] But if it does get past that layer, into an inner layer called the lamina propria, inflammation can start. Many other factors — such as infections, toxins, stress, and age — can also cause these tight junctions to break apart. The research is still unclear on the exact mechanisms of how this works, but we do know that food allergies and food intolerances play a major role.

Here are a few signs you have a leaky gut:

- Gas, bloating, diarrhea, or irritable bowel syndrome (IBS)
- Hormonal imbalances such as painful PMS or PCOS
- Diagnosis of an autoimmune disease such as rheumatoid arthritis, Hashimoto's thyroiditis, or celiac disease
- Diagnosis of chronic fatigue or fibromyalgia
- Depression, anxiety, ADD, or ADHD
- Skin issues such as acne, rosacea, or eczema
- Asthma
- Food allergies or food intolerances[9]

So what are common allergen triggers?

We are often sensitive to modern, convenient foods containing preservatives, pesticides, GMOs, and MSG. These substances can be hard for the digestive system to process, creating discomfort. We also know that certain foods like sugar, gluten, dairy, processed soy, peanuts, eggs, and corn can also be triggers for food sensitivities.

HOW CAN WE FIX IT?

How can we reduce inflammation? Well, it shouldn't come as a surprise by now that my answer is going to be mostly about your diet and lifestyle choices. And most of those choices are based on thousands of tiny decisions you make each day that are (whether or not you know it) either anti- or pro-inflammatory. What time will you wake up? What will you have for breakfast? What time will you eat? What does your morning routine look like? What kind of exercise will you do? What kind of dressing will you have on your salad? How long will you stay at work? What will you do when you get home to unwind? Small choices can have a BIG impact, and there are a few key factors that will help fend off chronic inflammation: mostly it's eating the right food, getting good shut-eye, and reducing stress.

Food

A 2013 landmark study called PREDIMED followed 7,447 people, aged 55 to 80 years old, who had diabetes, high blood pressure, or high cholesterol over the course of about five years; 57 percent of the study participants were women.[10] These individuals were put on a food plan similar to the Mediterranean diet, which included fruits, vegetables, fish, legumes, olive oil, certain nuts, and sofrito (a tomato sauce with garlic herbs and olive oil), and excluded processed foods of any kind—sugar, soda, spread fats like margarine, and red and processed meat.

After almost five years, there was a 30 percent difference in the heart attack/stroke rates of the two groups. Inflammatory markers were down, too, for those on the Mediterranean-type diet, and their telomere lengths were longer — meaning that they had "aged" less than those in the group not on the diet. What are telomeres, you ask? They are like the plastic tips on shoelaces — protective caps on the ends of DNA and protein that prevent them from fraying. Telomeres naturally shorten over the course of your life, but there is significant variation in how fast this happens. In short, a pro-inflammatory diet — characterized by a high intake of meat, refined (white) grains, added sugars, and foods rich in saturated and trans fats — increases the risk of telomere shortening, which eventually leads to earlier death. (Even though there was some controversy over the protocol of the study, its findings have held up over time.)

I was guilty of eating a very similar pro-inflammatory diet before my car accident. Although I considered myself a healthy eater since I had plenty of fruits and salads, I didn't realize that I was also consuming a lot of hidden processed foods and sugar. Starbucks lattes and granola bars were my staples. And having grown up in New York, bagels were one of my favorite meals on the go. All these types of foods can turn your gut into a factory for chronic, or "silent," inflammation. These foods increase the levels of blood sugar from processed carbohydrates or sugar and contribute to an increase in free radicals and pro-inflammatory cytokines, chemicals that kick off chronic inflammation in the body.

So I learned what foods were anti-inflammatory and started adding them into my diet, and I couldn't believe the difference I felt in a matter of a few days. I now know that making simple changes — that is, eliminating high fructose corn syrup, white sugar, gluten, and white flours — can lead to big benefits. We'll go into these dietary changes in more detail in chapter 8, but here's an overview of what's good to eat to lower inflammation and up your energy levels.

Add Fiber, Fiber, Fiber

Food is the best lever for change in your inflammatory state. Centenarians are known to follow a whole foods diet with tons of vegetables. So if you want to live that long, fiber is key. And vegetables in particular will give you more antioxidants and polyphenols, which can fight free radicals and can calm inflammation. If there's one thing I've learned from my research, it's that adding fiber is crucial to healing your gut and lowering inflammation. Most gut bacteria live in the distal colon — the last area in the intestines — so getting food there is key. But most food (protein, carbs, and fats) gets digested before reaching the distal colon. Fiber doesn't, so the good bacteria can feed on it when it reaches the distal colon.

Why is it important to feed that specific bacteria? Because these bacteria create short-chain fatty acids, which perform the vital function of calming the immune system and making it less reactive. These short-chain fatty acids signal more regulatory T cells, which help to prevent autoimmunity and allergies.

If we don't get enough fiber, the bacteria starve and start eating mucin, which is the lining between our intestinal cells and bacteria (which can lead to leaky gut). It's estimated that hunter-gatherer societies consumed upward of 200 grams of fiber daily, while the average modern American now gets just 15 grams a day. Yep, you read that right.

The best source is complex carbohydrates from fermentable plant fibers. So you should eat more cellulose fibers, present in the tough parts of veggies and fruits, like broccoli stalks, the bottom of asparagus, kale stems, and orange pulp. Vegetables contain hundreds to thousands of phytonutrients — literally plant hormones — that have hormone-balancing and anti-inflammatory effects (a twofer!) in the body. Vegetables as well as fruits also supply us with fiber that binds itself to old estrogen, thereby clearing it out of the system, leading to better overall hormonal equilibrium. This is great for both men and women who suffer from estrogen dominance.

Vegetables also supply prebiotic fibers that good bacteria feed on in the gut. This fiber is most abundantly found in asparagus, chicory root, leeks, onions, and garlic.

You will want to aim for at least three — but ideally up to nine — cups of vegetables a day. Start slowly with well-cooked vegetables twice a day (newbies to the plan may not be used to this much fiber, so cooking helps with digestion), and then gradually add more every day.

Cut Out Inflammatory Foods

While everyone is different and will react differently to different foods, for many people, foods like processed dairy, gluten, alcohol, processed snacks, omega-6 oils, and processed soy can incite inflammation and manipulate hormones. Without rigorous testing, it's hard to pinpoint where inflammation is coming from, but foodwise public enemy number one is sugar.

Ditch Sugar

Sugar and refined carbohydrates spark inflammation by deregulating glucose and insulin, leading to oxidative stress. In short, insulin resistance triggers the inflammation cascade. Sugar is the *most* inflammatory food you can eat. There are three types of sugar: fructose, glucose, and lactose. All naturally come from food, but our body metabolizes each of them differently. And fructose sugar has been shown to be the most inflammatory of the three. It's important to note that fructose is naturally found in fruits. The key word here is *naturally*. It's a problem when it's separated from the fruit and made into high fructose corn syrup. If you are eating whole fruit, its fructose does not have the same negative effects. Once you start reading labels, it's shocking how many foods contain fructose, including soda, candy, even flavored yogurt.

Reconsider Refined Flour and Gluten

The word "refined" in flour refers to a modification process where the bran and germ are removed, allowing products to stay on the shelf longer; however, this process also removes the naturally occurring vitamins, minerals, and dietary fiber. Similar to refined sugar, refined flours also deregulate insulin. Gluten is a protein contained in wheat. Gluten in particular is not only inflammatory because of its "sugar-like" properties when refined — it's also a gut irritant. (Celiac disease is an autoimmune reaction triggered by gluten.) Stick to whole grains (I like rye, sprouted whole grain, and barley), and, if gluten-free, buckwheat, quinoa, oats, and brown rice are all great choices.

Consider Ditching Dairy

I grew up on dairy (after all, milk did a body good, right?), and I loved my ice cream. But as a physician, I have been influenced by the science. I study and work with patients who have food allergies, intolerances, and immunology issues, and what I see in my practice is that for many people, through many different mechanisms, dairy is causing unwanted inflammation.

In adults, there are multiple mechanisms that make dairy inflammatory, depending upon the patient's genetic predisposition and many other factors. Some people aren't allergic but have an inflammatory response to dairy. A large percentage of people in the world are lactose intolerant, which means they aren't fully able to digest the milk proteins.

What is it about milk and dairy that makes us feel so bad? There are many problematic proteins in dairy, but casein, casomorphin, and butyrophilin are the main ones. In fact, T. Colin Campbell, author of *The China Study*, has linked increased casein intake with increased incidence of cancer.

Because dairy can be so inflammatory, if you suspect that inflammation is your primary issue, I recommend cutting dairy out of your diet for one month. If after one month you don't feel better, you can add it back to your diet. If dairy doesn't bother you, feel free to have it.

That said, please don't consume conventional milk or fat-free options. One dairy option is raw or fermented, full-fat dairy in small amounts (up to total 80–120 calories a day). Raw and full fat is great because it is closest to the way it comes out of the cow. Pasteurization, which is a heating process that kills bacteria, also reduces the milk's nutritional value. Do be careful, as raw milk can carry dangerous bacteria like listeria, salmonella, and other microbes that can cause food poisoning. So investigate the quality of the source and the local laws in your state about raw milk consumption, and if you are pregnant, it's best to steer clear of unpasteurized milk altogether.

Try going dairy-free for a month, and if you *do* feel better, take that into account — it means dairy is likely causing inflammation and you may want to cut it from your diet. If you don't see any differences after a month without dairy, add in fermented, full-fat, or raw dairy in small amounts and see how you feel.

Take Vitamins D and B

Vitamin D is *key* in lowering inflammation, and it plays a significant role in gastrointestinal health. Vitamin D works like a hormone in the body, constantly turning off and on hundreds of genes, and therefore influencing our health.

Unfortunately, vitamin D deficiency is really common, and, worse, the World Health Organization has found an association between low vitamin D and inflammation-related diseases. There are actually D receptors in our teeth, salivary glands, esophagus, and stomach, and low vitamin D levels are linked to slow stomach emptying and bile production, putting the trifecta in flux — inciting inflammation and triggering hormone disruption. Not only that, research suggests that vitamin D deficiency is a common denominator in many critical illnesses. For example, through research we know that children with low vitamin D are prone to more diseases such as asthma and allergies.

You might be wondering where you're supposed to get your vitamin D if you're not eating dairy. Although you can obtain D from the sun, it's often not enough, especially if you are dark-skinned. Though some foods like oily fish and fortified milk contain vitamin D, I recommend supplementing with at least 5,000 IU a day.

Another vitamin that is linked to inflammation is vitamin B. There is still much to be determined about how vitamin B can help, but in recent studies, B vitamins such as B_6, folate (B_9), and B_{12} can lower your levels of homocysteine — an inflammatory protein already linked to Alzheimer's and heart disease. While the true effect of B vitamins in large randomized studies remains to be seen, B vitamins also seem to bring down another inflammatory factor called C-reactive protein. All in all, it looks like it's a safe bet to add this onto your what-to-eat list.

Eat Healthy Fats (and Avoid the Harmful Kind)

Just a few decades ago, we were told to avoid fats of most kinds. But that thinking is outdated — it turns out some fats are very necessary for our overall health and are essential to consume. But, of course, not all fats are created equal.

A good rule of thumb about food is to remember that the closer we eat to the earth, the healthier it is for us. So consider fats by how natural they are: coconuts, avocados, olive oil (a mainstay of the Mediterranean diet), and other healthy sources of saturated fat boost female hormones and testosterone and help promote good (HDL) cholesterol. Cholesterol is needed for the formation of healthy cell membranes and is a precursor to all steroid hormones (progesterone, estrogen, FSH, etc.). We can't have proper hormonal balance without adequate amounts of fats. Steer clear of fats that include highly processed oils like vegetable oils, peanut oil, canola oil, soybean oil, cottonseed oil, sunflower oil, margarine, shortening, or "spreads," all of which are high in inflammatory omega-6 fats.

Adding oily fish and/or fish oil, which contain polyunsaturated omega-3 fats, to your diet is another way to help balance your hormones and lower inflammation; if you're vegan, algae oil is a great way to get omega 3s along with (to a lesser extent) chia seeds, flax, and walnuts. I actually prefer algae oil over fish oil since I know I am steering clear of any possible toxins and PCBs.

Avoid All-Day Caffeine

Excessive caffeine raises your cortisol and slows down your thyroid. Plus, it aggravates acid reflux and gut disorders. The key word here is *excessive*. That's not to say that you can't have a cup of coffee or tea. Plus, depending on your genetic makeup, you may be a better caffeine metabolizer than others. But when you're aggressively trying to fix your hormones, gut, and inflammation levels, try a trial of reduced or zero caffeine. And avoid any intake after noon, when it can interfere with your circadian rhythm.

Take Probiotics — but Not the Kind You Think

You've probably heard of probiotics — live "good" bacteria that are in certain foods like yogurt — and how they can keep your gut healthy. But did you know that the good bacteria in your gut help with inflammation, too? You want that good bacteria to grow and thrive.

Be careful in choosing your probiotic, though, as the supplement industry is notoriously underregulated. In fact, one study tested 14 commercial probiotics and found that only one contained the exact species stated on the label. That's why I recommend focusing on naturally probiotic foods first — like pickles, fermented vegetables, sauerkraut, kimchi, miso, natto, tempeh, kefir (nondairy), and apple cider vinegar — before turning to pills. Make sure you get your probiotic foods from the refrigerated section of the grocery store; otherwise the probiotics will no longer be live.

Add Adaptogens

The majority of India's population follows Ayurvedic medicine, either exclusively or in combination with conventional Western medicine. Ayurvedic medicine — an ancient Indian practice more than three thousand years old — has a more holistic take on the body, viewing our health as rooted in the interconnectedness of the body, mind, and spirit. We in the West are slowly seeing the benefits of basic Ayurvedic doctrines, paramount being the use of "adaptogen" herbs for healing. (Adaptogen refers to a plant's ability to adapt to its environment and exterior stress to survive.) When I was transforming my body, I found a combination of these herbs to be really helpful.

Herbs such as rhodiola, ashwagandha, ginseng, phosphatidylserine, and maca help strengthen and stabilize the body, thereby mollifying the impact of stress. Adaptogens also improve the entire body's resistance to stress (not just a particular organ or system) and create balance and harmony in the body, helping to reduce chronic inflammation. They are also traditionally used for digestive issues like constipation, as they are anti-inflammatory and can help calm the nervous and digestive systems and relieve stress in the body, promoting homeostasis. They can aid the body's physical and mental focus, decreasing what is called *ama* in Ayurvedic medicine — toxic waste — and the overall health of digestion.

Maca, in particular, is high in minerals and fatty acids, and it is especially good for hormone harmony. Many women notice less PMS, increased fertility, and improved skin when they incorporate maca into their diet, while men notice increased sperm production, higher libido, and better sleep. Bonus: it tastes great in smoothies. Ashwagandha and rhodiola improve thyroid and adrenal function, creating systemic balance and increased energy.

What Are Ashwagandha and Rhodiola?

Ashwagandha (if you were wondering how to pronounce it, you are not alone: it's pronounced ˌä-shwə-ˈgän-də) is an ancient Ayurvedic herb that has been long prescribed to strengthen the immune system and support physical, mental, and emotional health. It also has adaptogenic, anti-inflammatory, and stress-relieving properties.

Here's a short list of the many great properties of ashwagandha:

- It's anti-inflammatory. (Yes, I know it is a nightshade, but that should *not* be a problem for most.)
- It's an adaptogen, meaning it protects the body against chronic stress.
- It relaxes the central nervous system.
- It protects against free radicals, meaning it helps fight cancer.
- It boosts the immune system.
- It reduces anxiety and depression; stabilizes mood.
- It improves learning memory and mental sharpness.

Rhodiola is also an adaptogenic herb traditionally used as a tonic for fatigue, poor attention span, decreased memory, and increased vitality. It is also good for stress, inflammation, immunity, and the other benefits listed below.

Rhodiola is good for the following:

- Reducing fatigue (especially from physical or mental "burnout")
- Relieving stress
- Repairing damage from oxygen deprivation
- Providing antioxidants
- Enhancing immune function
- Increasing sexual energy
- Helping physical performance
- Aiding mental performance
- Reducing inflammation

I like to use adaptogens during any period of time when I feel like I require extra help with energy and inflammation, but then I go off them for a week to reassess if I still need them. This way, I minimize my supplement taking, but I still use them for support as needed. (I always go with the adage that less is more when it comes to supplements.)

GET MORE SHUT-EYE

I have to admit that before my accident, I often tried to be "super-mom" and do it all—on six hours or less of sleep a night. And I am sure I am not the only woman guilty of this! Lack of sleep makes the body ripe for infection, while getting adequate sleep has an anti-inflammatory effect. A 2010 study from the Emory School of Medicine in Atlanta found that short sleep durations and poor sleep quality are associated with higher levels of inflammation markers.[11] In fact, individuals who reported six or fewer hours of sleep had the highest levels of inflammatory hormones and changes in blood vessel function. (We get much more into sleep in chapter 8.)

REMOVE STRESS

Well, that's impossible, I know, but how about trying to limit your stress levels? Until recently, it was relatively unclear why stress has such a heavy influence on disease and health, but we know now that chronic psychological stress influences the body's inflammatory response because stress genetically alters immune cells to poise them to fight infection or trauma.

Chronically elevated cortisol could be the hormone that's sabotaging your energy trifecta — even if you're doing everything else right. Even naturally thin people have to worry about cortisol. Researchers at Yale University, for example, found that slender women who had high cortisol were more likely to have excess abdominal fat (what they called "stress belly").[12]

I have said it before, and I'll say it again before the book is done: stress is one of the worst aggravators of inflammation. Cortisol was my personal nemesis — limited sleep, too much coffee, stressful days at work and with the kids, and long, hard cardio workouts threw me into a crisis. For me, getting cortisol under control with sleep, meditation, and yoga was the biggest step I took in fixing my energy trifecta. Surprisingly, creative outlets like writing, volunteering, and teaching also really helped me tap into those feel-good chemicals that counteract cortisol.

Making time in your schedule to include moments of mindfulness and stillness really does make a difference. Mindfulness is in fact the newest component of any wellness plan (yet it is an ancient practice). New studies indicate that the immune system is directly connected to the brain, therefore lowering inflammation can help treat diseases like depression and anxiety. This also lends more credence to the fact that daily mindfulness/meditation is anti-inflammatory. Yoga, walking, and even reading a good book can all help bring down those levels.

It's a no-brainer that getting out in nature and breathing in fresh air and experiencing quiet is good for the soul. There's something about being away from all the stimulation of urban existence and wrapping oneself in natural scenery that creates a sense of calm and relaxes the central nervous system. Some research suggests that direct contact with the earth — being barefoot in the grass or on a beach — affects white blood cells, cytokines, and other molecules that regulate inflammation. This grounding in nature can help improve sleep, regulate cortisol, and alleviate stress. Though grounding is literally touching skin to earth, physical exposure to nature can produce the same calmative effect that may physiologically reduce inflammation. The feeling of the earth under your feet is not only soothing, but you may be absorbing electrons from the earth through the soles of your feet that impact inflammatory response.

Here are other ways to keep inflammation at bay:

Exercise the Right Way

Watch your exercise. No pain, no gain, right? Actually, wrong. In the past, I was a glutton for punishment when it came to exercise, so this one was hard for me. But I backed off of doing long cardio sessions five to six days a week and started doing yoga and shorter-burst training to prevent that chronic cortisol elevation. I still like to go for runs from time to time, but I don't go as hard or as often as I did before. Shockingly, I actually got in better shape after I reduced my cardio.

Pushing yourself to the limit every day on top of a stressful lifestyle can lower your thyroid function and increase cortisol and inflammation. However, interval training (a combination of low- and high-intensity exercises) increases your HGH (human growth hormone) and slows down aging. (We'll talk more about working out in the WTF plan in chapter 8.)

Check In with Your Modern Environment

We have talked about endocrine disrupters, or hormone disrupters, in the last chapter, and these guys hit the trifecta hard. Not only do they affect your hormones, but they also have adverse developmental, reproductive, neurological, and immune effects. And they can cause inflammation and gut flora imbalance.

Hormone disrupters are everywhere, unfortunately. We only know about the tip of the iceberg with regard to chemical endocrine disrupters. The comprehensive list contains about 870 disrupters, and more are discovered all the time! But what you can do is be cognizant and educate yourself about the most harmful ones. At the very least, try to avoid lead, parabens, phthalates, and bisphenol A (BPA). Common offenders include plastics, air fresheners, dishwashing soap, laundry detergent, cleansers and cleaners, cosmetics, deodorants, toothpaste, shaving gel, and lotions. Check labels and use resources like ewg.org.

Start small: Try to swap out some of your most-used products for ones that aren't disruptive. Check out natural toothpastes without fluoride, sweeteners, and additives. In the shower, use a soap that is natural like Dove, and shampoos and conditioners from natural-product companies like Babo Botanicals, Honest, or Beautycounter. There are more and more companies that espouse having only all-natural ingredients, so just make sure the products you use are unscented, uncolored, and without parabens.

This is my goal for you: to feel your most vibrant and energetic — and reducing inflammation is key to that equation. And so while inflammation is not so easy to detect, it is amazing how small dietary and lifestyle changes can help *decrease* inflammation and *increase* your energy levels — perhaps so much so that you can rock those sexy high heels as you race to your next meeting, not to mention giving you a longer and healthier life to wear those killer heels.

5

Gut Reaction

I HATE TO SAY IT, but I think my Frappuccinos are killing me," Emily, a busy LA designer, confessed as she sat across from me in my office.

I wouldn't have put it in such dire terms, but unfortunately she was correct. Those yummy drinks were hurting her health. She had come to my practice a month before, complaining of a mixed bag of seemingly unrelated symptoms: overall fatigue, bloating, and an odd case of rashes. She had already seen my husband, a board-certified gastroenterologist, who, after giving her a colonoscopy and doing lab work, was baffled and sent her to me. As a doctor, he knew something more was wrong, but he was at the end of what traditional medicine could offer her.

After some testing, including an IgE food allergy test that came back negative, I had her keep a food diary of what she ate and drank for a week.

I had a feeling that what she was eating was causing her problems. Hippocrates, considered the Father of Medicine, nailed it more than two thousand years ago when he wrote: "All disease begins in the gut." (He must have been onto something, because he lived to about ninety.) I'd like to add an addendum to this: all energy begins in the gut, too.

When Emily returned to my office with her journal, I read through her scribbled notes and could see that she was careful to eat healthily throughout the day: yogurt in the morning, a healthy salad at lunch, and chicken or fish for dinner. No sneaking treats in between meals or overindulging in carbs. One thing stuck out, though: her 3 p.m. "please don't let me crash" Starbucks Mocha Frappuccino she bought nearly every day. Don't be fooled: this isn't just coffee. There are 52 grams of sugar in a grande Mocha Frap. The daily recommendation for women by the American Heart Association is *half* that. She was spending a lot of money on making herself sick.

A lot of great studies have come out in the last ten years that have revealed so much in terms of how our gut plays into our overall health. It is really important to understand how our health is intricately connected to what we eat. Food can't be the be-all and end-all cure of disease, but it sure can help keep it at bay.

What's more, not only is the gut (and its bacteria) key to keeping us healthy by absorbing nutrients we need and discarding viruses and other foreign invaders, but this delicate ecosystem made up of billions and billions of microorganisms supports our immune system and, I will argue, helps control our energy.

THE INFLAMED GUT

There has been a lot of exciting new research about how hormones live and breathe in our gut, and studies that show that microbes are intimately related to our immune system. We also now know that 70–80 percent of the immune system lives in the gut. These microbes are the first thing that food, viruses, bacteria, or toxins see when they travel through the GI tract. The gut is in constant communication with our hormones as well, since the gastrointestinal cells have receptors that sense any sort of hormonal changes. It has been said that 90 percent of hormone imbalances can be traced back to gut health.[1]

Dr. Justin Sonnenburg — associate professor in microbiology at Stanford University, coauthor of *The Good Gut,* and leading researcher in the gut microbiota — has said, "These microbes in our gut are dictating the set point of our immune system throughout our body. They can impact things like respiratory infections, how well we respond to a vaccine, how rapidly an autoimmune disease can progress. So I think this insight that so much of our immune system is in our gut is really profound, and it's important to recognize that this not only impacts what's going on in the gut but throughout our entire body."[2]

There is a fascinating, ongoing conversation in our gut between our immune system and the gut microbes, which together block out pathogens, food particles, and toxins. But this conversation can be cut short or compromised, and how this happens is pretty simple, really. When we eat food, our gut bacteria sense the food and send a message to our immune cells. Our gut bacteria and immune cells put the food we eat into two camps: foods they are familiar with and thus "approve" (like some human version of quality control) or something they're not familiar with that is "rejected" and labeled an invader.

To better understand this, let's first take a look at something that the gut recognizes. Think of the last piece of "whole" food you have eaten — say, a blueberry. Not in ice cream or a muffin, just a simple, delicious, summer-fresh blueberry. Pretty darn healthy choice! Anyway, that berry will travel to the stomach and into your intestines, where a whole army of bacteria examines the fruit and determines what our body can take from it. In a complex communication that we don't yet fully understand, that quality-control system recognizes the berry, and the gut communicates back and forth with the immune system to keep it moving. The berry is "approved" and is extracted of all its good nutrients, which are then transported to where they need to go via the bloodstream.

Now let's see what happens when Emily has that Frappuccino. As she drinks it and it goes through her digestive system, the gut bacteria may not recognize all of the drink's many ingredients or may recognize some of them — like the milk, sugar, and flavored syrups (and don't forget the whipped cream) — but determine them to be toxic. What sets off these alarms? Any processed food, like chemicals in the syrup or even in the milk. The gut bacteria will then "talk" to the immune system, warning it that something foreign has entered the system. The immune cells flood the area, removing all the bad stuff, taking in the calories and sugar, carbohydrates, and any protein. This dairy or preservative, depending on the person, can irritate the gut lining, which sets off another set of alarm bells to the immune system, which in turn gets confused and sends reinforcements to that area. And this can repeat if, let's say, you wolf down a delicious muffin with that Frappuccino. When the processed ingredients in that muffin reach your digestive system, the food again looks unfamiliar and the immune system may send another troop to check it out. This constant assault to the response system can create acute inflammation in your gut. And if you don't let the system repair and rest, and it's working late into the night while you are losing valuable shut-eye, your gut lining, bacteria, gut, and immune system will continue down the path of exhaustion. They just can't catch a break, and chronic inflammation will set in. If you continue to eat crap that is processed and the body is not set up to recognize the ingredients, let alone extract anything nutritious from them, you are in for a big surprise. You have created an environment where the body's response team is exhausted and nothing gets repaired because it's dealing with crisis after crisis.

And that is basically the crux of our modern diet. Add into the mix chemicals, toxins like alcohol, artificial additives and colors, and pollution, and we have the perfect-storm scenario for an inflamed gut.

So if day in, day out you eat like this and then add to it a genetic predisposition that compromises the immune system or if the gut bacteria aren't as varied as they should be, the system will break down, not be able to digest the food, and set off a host of problems. End result: fatigue, bloating, autoimmune diseases. Excess sugars and other toxins will cause bacteria to break down, as do antibiotics, NSAIDs, and glyphosate. Eventually, all this will damage the gut by creating cracks or holes in the intestinal lining, in which bacteria can "leak" into the bloodstream and can cause widespread inflammation and even trip a wire with the immune system. This condition is known as "leaky gut."

Then the inevitable bloat comes on, and you become tired as f*@k. Emily had such symptoms, and I believe she had a leaky gut that if left untreated could go on to create serious digestive issues, skin problems, and other major chronic conditions that will chisel away at her health. Worse, many GI experts are convinced that a good number of patients who have leaky gut will likely progress to more severe GI conditions, some of which are irreversible.

YOUR GARDEN OF GUT FLORA

Now that we know how the immune system works in tandem with the gut, let's dig a bit deeper. Did you know there are an estimated 100 *trillion* bacteria in your gut? In other words, we have five to ten times more bacterial cells than human cells in our bodies.[3]

This microbiome has long been part of us, going back thousands and thousands of years. The biome contains good and bad bacteria. This may come as a surprise, because typically we portray bacteria as bad guys that try to make us sick, and we fight them off with antibiotics and antibacterial products. And have you noticed that pretty much any cleaning product touts itself as "antibacterial" these days? Soaps, hand sanitizers, wipes, even toothpaste claim to ward off these nasty buggers.

But groundbreaking research in the past several years has shown that some bacteria are not only good for us but necessary for our health.[4] And as long as the good bacteria outweigh the bad, you will enjoy high energy levels, a healthy digestive tract, and a clear, focused mind as bacteria do their job and work for us 24/7. What exactly do they do for us? Some bacteria produce enzymes to break down foods, while others produce vitamins and vital compounds like the feel-good neurotransmitter serotonin. (The idea of a "gut feeling" is no joke: 95 percent of serotonin and other neurotransmitters are produced in the gut! An imbalanced gut microbiome can lead to a host of immune, mood, and energy issues.) Some bacteria regulate the metabolism, which tells you when you are hungry, full, and when you *need* that 4 p.m. snack. Gut flora does so much for our immune system, and we are really only beginning to understand how to optimize this microbiome to maximize our health.

Unfortunately, recent studies show that the average American gut microbiome is not as diverse and plentiful as it was for our ancestors or even for people in non-Western cultures.[5] There is a growing belief that our Western culture, diet, and lifestyle have caused a decrease in that wonderful diversity of our microbiota. Recent studies had demonstrated that there is a connection between the decrease in the microbiome's bacterial content and the increase of obesity, autoimmune and gastrointestinal diseases, and other conditions in Western countries. In another recent study, the Western microbiome has shown a decrease of some types of bacteria that process complex and vegetal fibers in the intestine as opposed to non-Westerners' or prehistoric microbiomes.[6] The supposition is that the Western diet is higher in fat and sugar and lower in fiber intake. A sedentary lifestyle doesn't help, nor do our incessant, nearly OCD-level hygiene habits and the widespread use of antibiotics. We are safer in this modern lifestyle, for sure, but there is the downside to this safety of losing that delicate gut microbiota balance.

And when you don't have enough gut bacteria talking to your immune system, you get a breakdown that can lead to leaky gut as well as other chronic conditions and diseases.[7] So we need a healthy population of bacteria to keep your body functioning optimally.

Leaky Gut

What is a leaky gut, exactly? While the medical community continues to debate whether or not it is a real condition, there is increasingly more science that confirms its existence, at least when it comes to intestinal permeability. Think of your gut as a thick, hardy tube that runs from your mouth all the way to your anus. It's pretty resilient — it needs to be because its job is to help keep anything foreign out of rest of the body. Nothing is supposed to get into our organs and bloodstream without our immune system saying it's okay. This tube prevents foreign material (i.e., food) from getting into the rest of the body and bloodstream, while allowing microorganisms and nutrients through. Yet chronic inflammation can cause gaps or holes in the gut lining that let larger particles through, by what is called "intestinal permeability." Or in layperson's terms, leaky gut. The gut lining can also be damaged by toxins, foods, medications, and stress. These particles are treated as foreign invaders — like a virus — and are attacked.

What Can Cause Leaky Gut?

- Processed foods containing fillers, stabilizers, and other chemical products
- Foods that contain GMOs (of course, this is up for debate, but corn and soybean are two of the most common)
- Excess salt and sugar
- Food sensitivities to things like dairy and gluten
- Certain medications like ibuprofen and antibiotics
- Environmental toxins
- Beauty products
- Air pollution
- Plastics and metals
- Cleaning products

Factors surrounding birth and childhood can also make people more susceptible to leaky gut. Some predisposing factors are having been born by C-section and being formula fed as a baby, as both of these can disrupt the balance of gut bacteria.

An untreated leaky gut can lead to a slew of diseases, including IBS, Crohn's, cancer, autism, as well as autoimmune and metabolic disorders like obesity and diabetes. Have you had issues with bloating, indigestion, cramping, or gas? Food allergies and intolerances that are causing you to bloat or have abdominal discomfort can be a sign of leaky gut. There is also a theory that leaky gut may not cause gut symptoms. For example, a majority of people with "leaky gut" do not experience digestive distress; rather the issue manifests itself in other seemingly unrelated ways, including skin problems, brain fog, anxiety, autoimmune disease, and joint pain.[8] No matter what, leaky gut, even though not an official medical diagnosis, is something to avoid at all costs.

The Interconnectedness of Your Gut and Brain

We talked a little bit about how we are just discovering how the brain is connected to our gut and how the gut can affect metabolism, the immune system, and brain health. We know, for instance, that the brain and gut are literally connected by the myenteric plexus — a network of nerve fibers and neuron cells influenced by signals from the brain — which lines our intestinal walls. In this sense, the gut is an integral part of the nervous system, so the brain can easily affect gut function. There is growing scientific evidence that your brain detects when your gut is "inflamed," and resulting feelings of sadness or anxiety can arise. Gut bacteria may also produce molecules that make us crave sugar and/or feel worried.

Stress and emotions regulate gut health and vice versa: anxiety, stress, and depression can influence digestion, manifesting in stomachaches, nutrient malabsorption, and GI issues. Unbalanced gut flora and leaky gut can influence neurotransmitters, creating depression, mood disorders, irritability, ADHD, brain fog, and anxiety or over-exhaustion. Research is even drawing connections between gut health and serious conditions like autism, diabetes, and Alzheimer's disease.

There are two problems that the immune system can encounter: overactivity and underactivity. You don't want either. Underactivity is a very serious disorder that is usually detected at birth; those who have it may not make it to adulthood. We'll be talking about an overactive immune system that is often labeled as an autoimmune disorder. Autoimmunity leads to food and environmental allergies, asthma, eczema, and conditions like Crohn's, Hashimoto's, and diabetes. An underactive immune system causes you to get sick often or makes you more susceptible to infections, viruses, and fungal or yeast infections. Because the gut and the immune system are so intimately connected, this is why a lot of autoimmune issues improve or disappear once you reset the gut.

QUIZ: DO YOU HAVE A GUT FLORA IMBALANCE?

Your gut is made up of microbial cells and bacteria, both good and bad. As long as the good outweighs the bad, there is equilibrium, and not only a healthy digestive tract, but also a well-running body that keeps you going like the Energizer Bunny. How do you know if you have an imbalance? Do you have

- Digestive issues: bloating, constipation, indigestion, etc.
- Depression/anxiety
- Brain fog
- Fatigue
- Skin issues: eczema, psoriasis, athlete's foot
- Metabolic problems: inability to lose weight, weight gain, diabetes
- Allergies
- Asthma
- An autoimmune disease
- Frequent illnesses

If you answer yes to two or more of these symptoms, then you likely have some form of gut flora imbalance. (If you do, don't panic — the WTF plan is designed to help you!)

As a reminder, here are some common causes of gut flora imbalance:

- Antibiotics
- Birth control
- NSAIDs (aspirin, ibuprofen, anti-inflammatories)
- Diets high in refined sugar and carbs and processed foods
- Diets low in fermentable fibers (whole grains, fruits, vegetables)
- Chronic stress
- Neurological disorders and conditions
- Over-sanitation/over-cleansing

The Woman Has Guts

New studies have shown that gut microbiota are key in the regulation of our estrogen levels. In fact, there's even a specific group of microbes dedicated to estrogen, known as the estrobolome. This estrobolome consists of microbes capable of metabolizing estrogen. Dysbiosis — a microbiome imbalance — can either reduce or increase the amount of estrogen produced.[9] Too much or too little estrogen can wreak havoc on the body and increase the risk of developing estrogen-related diseases such as endometriosis, PCOS, and breast cancer. In postmenopausal women, there's an increased risk of obesity, cardiovascular disease, and osteoporosis if there is any sort of dysfunction.[10] So, ladies, let's keep those estrogen levels balanced, shall we?

HOW DO WE KEEP THAT GARDEN LUSH?

There are many natural ways to keep our microbiome vibrant and healthy. Let's talk about what we can eat and what we should avoid to do just that; let's get the bad guys out of the way first.

What to Avoid

The number one culprit causing problems in the gut is processed sugar. Don't eat anything with added sugar if you can help it. I am talking 5 grams or less — much less than the American Heart Association's recommended allowance of 25 grams, which is way too high in my opinion. Why? Sugar nourishes pathogenic (or bad) bacteria, yeast, and fungus in the gut. It's literally food for the WRONG bacteria. It's absorbed early in the GI tract and gives you quick energy and then a big crash. To further this point, artificial sweeteners like aspartame should be avoided at all costs. (High-quality stevia — a natural extract from plants — is an acceptable sugar alternative.) Fruit is also okay, along with naturally occurring sugars in raw foods like sweet potato.

Antibiotics are something else to consider when it comes to our gut health. They are taken to kill bad bacteria that are making us sick, but they end up killing not just the bad bugs, but the good bacteria, too. Studies show that antibiotics "derange" the microbiome, even causing some species to go extinct. It's very difficult to recover from this "nuclear bomb" to your gut. So if you must take antibiotics, make sure they're absolutely necessary. To replenish your body after a round of antibiotics, you want to make sure you eat good, whole foods, especially prebiotic and probiotic foods (no supplements). (The same concept can go for popular hand sanitizers today: excessive cleanliness can also affect gut health. Covid-19 or no Covid-19, overuse of hand sanitizers, cleaning products, and bleach severely damages the microbiome. If any of you have kids or are around kids, encourage them to play with and around dirt. Although this is not shown as clearly in studies, dirt is good for adults as well for the same reasons. Try NOT to over-sanitize!)

Virus Protection in a Post-Covid-19 World

For years, doctors and health experts have warned about
over-sanitizing, as it has been shown to kill good bacteria
along with the bad, and thus jeopardizes our healthy gut flora
(remember, at least 70 percent of our immune system is in
our gut). That mentality went out the window when Covid-19
hit in early 2020. Since the disease was so novel, the scientific
community had little to go on in terms of how it spread —
only that it was much more contagious than the flu. So the
public was told to wear masks, wipe down everything that we
touched, stay at home. Suddenly we couldn't sanitize enough:
we became toilet-paper-hoarding, Lysol-by-the-case-buying,
mask-wearing isolationists scared to leave our homes until the
worst of it had passed. The question is: How can we keep our
gut health in check in a post-pandemic world? My answer:
common sense. While we have to remain vigilant, overdoing
it can still create a catch-22, because over-sanitizing and
washing can kill the good gut bacteria that help our immune
system combat viruses like Covid-19. I prefer actually
washing hands with soap and water (the twenty-second rule)
over hand sanitizers as sanitizers can often contain toxic
ingredients. And of course, eat the right foods so that you can
create more good gut bacteria than you kill off. Keep being
vigilant and stay up on the latest news about how any new
viruses may spread.

There are other important things to avoid to maintain your gut
health:

NSAIDs: Nonsteroidal anti-inflammatory drugs — that is, ibuprofen and aspirin — are known to damage the gut lining and should
also be avoided to prevent leaky gut.

Conventional dairy: Any store-bought, non-organic milk, cheese,
or yogurt is also in the no-go zone. Dairy can easily irritate our microbiome, especially if you have undiagnosed dairy sensitivities or

allergies; studies link milk with inflammation, which we now know is linked to chronic disease.

Processed foods: Usually anything in a bag, box, or can, with more than three ingredients (think Doritos or even ketchup), is another major cause of our gut dysfunction. The more a food is processed, the more likely it is to be seen as a foreign invader or threat by the GI tract.

Gluten: The protein found in wheat is often present in processed foods, and it is a common trigger for a leaky gut for genetically susceptible people, even those who don't have a condition called celiac disease, which is a more severe intolerance to gluten.

GMOs: There's lots of talk about the effect of GMOs on the gut. But as of yet there is no convincing evidence to make it a primary recommendation for removal.

WHAT TO EAT

It's All About Fiber

If there is one thing I have learned from my research, it's that eating more fiber is key to healing the gut. It's literally food for your gut bacteria. Hunter-gatherer societies were able to rack up to 200 grams of fiber a day, while we get a measly 15 grams with our typical modern-day diet. We just don't get enough fiber to keep our gut in a healthy place.

As explained briefly in chapter 4, most gut bacteria live in the distal colon, the last stop in the intestines, so getting food there is key. And yet most of the nutrients in the food we eat — namely, protein, carbs, and fats — get digested before reaching the distal colon. Fiber, on the other hand, does not, so the good bacteria can feed on it when it reaches the distal colon. It's important to feed that specific bacteria in the colon because they create short-chain fatty acids (SFAs). These short-chain fatty acids signal more regulatory T cells, which help to prevent autoimmunity and allergies. We absorb SFAs, and they perform the vital function of calming the immune system and making it less reactive. What if we don't get enough fiber? The bacteria starve and start eating mucin, which is the lining between our intestinal cells and bacteria. And there you have it, the dreaded leaky gut.

So where do we get more fiber? The best source is complex carbohydrates from fermentable plant fibers: prebiotics, which are foods likely to encourage the growth of good bacteria, or probiotics, already present in the gut. We read so much about probiotics, but prebiotics are like food for probiotics, making them more effective. To get more prebiotics, you should eat more cellulose fibers, present in the tough parts of veggies and fruit (think of broccoli stalks, the bottom of asparagus, kale stems, and orange pulp).

The following foods are especially rich in prebiotics:

- Yams
- Potatoes
- Other tubers
- Ginger
- Leeks (green and white parts)
- Fibrous parts of fruit and vegetables
- Legumes/beans

The Wonders of Fermented Foods

Bone broth has enjoyed an amazing resurgence in popularity recently by Instagram influencers and health advocates alike, and we can trace its roots back to our man Hippocrates, who apparently peddled it to his patients as a remedy. But let me be blunt for a minute: bone broth is overrated and overhyped. There are a lot of claims out there that bone broth is a power-packed low-calorie, high-protein food rich in collagen and other essential minerals and vitamins to aid in joint health, anti-inflammation, weight loss, among an ever-growing list of benefits. But just because it's trendy and your favorite celeb/athlete/Instagrammer is doing it doesn't mean it is the magic elixir that many claim it to be.

There is little evidence, in fact, that getting protein, collagen, and vitamins this way is more beneficial to the body than other food groups. Advocates rejoice in its gut-bacteria benefits. But while some studies show that potential in rats, we don't know if this is replicated in humans.[11] There are plenty of other benefits that bone broth advocates espouse that can be found easily in plants. Take, for instance, kale: a cup of raw kale contains much more calcium (90 mg) than a cup of bone broth (9–14 mg). A cup of chickpeas has a little more protein (11 grams) compared to bone broth (10 grams).

So, my opinion? Eh. I say stick to what has been proven to work: plant-based food rich in prebiotic fiber. For an extra jolt of gut-enriching nutrients, reach for fermented foods and drinks that give you "ready-made" probiotic bacteria.

FERMENTED AND CULTURED FOODS:
- Sauerkraut
- Kimchi
- Miso
- Natto
- Tempeh

FERMENTED DAIRY (IF YOU CAN TOLERATE IT):
- Yogurt
- Kefir
- Cottage cheese
- Sour cream/crème fraîche

No beer, sorry.

Probiotics

Probiotic — or fermented — foods provide a great amount of nutrients and phytochemicals.

You may have seen celeb-laced ads plugging yogurts and other probiotic drinks — it's a thing, apparently. There are tons of probiotics out there and many with accompanying studies that support their efficacy — but, ultimately, most are not known to have any beneficial effects and are thus a waste of your money. Commercial probiotics are hugely underregulated, so there is no measure of what is enough or too much. Label claims are often inaccurate, as is the amount of bacteria the probiotics are said to contain. In fact, it's nearly impossible to know just what you're getting when you buy probiotics. One study tested 14 commercial probiotics and found that only one contained the exact species listed on the label.[12] Plus, when you take in certain probiotics without changing your diet or lifestyle, it's basically like putting cattle on a barren land.

So why use them at all? You can effectively reap the benefits of probiotics by drinking kombucha or coconut kefir, fermented drinks that contain natural probiotics, which you can actually make yourself with kefir grains. If that sounds like too big an undertaking, KeVita is a great brand.

BONUS GUT SUPERFOODS:
- Coconut
- Digestive enzymes
- L glutamine
- Aloe vera
- Apple cider vinegar
- Turmeric
- CoQ10
- Magnesium
- Water first thing in the morning and 20 minutes before eating

But remember, all of these are extra. The best thing you can do is master the basics, particularly "getting more dirt" to strengthen and diversify your microbiome — and of course follow my WTF plan, which stresses eating good probiotic fiber and prebiotics.

OTHER WAYS TO TEND TO THAT GARDEN OF FLORA

Sleep, stress control, and intermittent fasting all help repair and reboot the gut. Why sleep? It is the *only* proven way to repair and reboot the immune system and the gut. I will be honest. If you want to heal your gut, reset your hormones, and shed some weight, you will need more rest than most. Most people who are going through this reset get the best results with a few days of restful sleep (turn off that alarm!). This tends to be more than eight hours. In fact, I need around nine hours!

Stress also has a negative effect on the gut. When you are stressed, you release hormones called CRFs, or corticotropin-releasing factors. These peptides are the signaling molecules of stress, and they are responsible for coordinating the body's response to stress. CRFs have a potent effect on the gut. They can lead to increased inflammation, gut permeability, visceral hypersensitivity, perception to pain, and gut motility. These hormones also cause the hypothalamic-pituitary-adrenal axis (HPA) to eventually stimulate the secretion of cortisol from the adrenal glands. Research in mice has found that exposure to stress led to an overgrowth of certain types of bacteria, while simultaneously reducing microbial diversity in the large intestine of stressed mice.

Keep the Garden Growing

Here is my takeaway for the long term:
1. Minimize sugar, keeping your intake of "treats" to around 10–15 percent or 200 calories (such as 1–2 servings of dark chocolate chips).
2. EAT FIBER EVERY DAY. *Don't* count calories — count fiber.
3. Eat more fermented, fibrous foods. (Have I mentioned fiber?) If you aren't able to consume fermented foods, take probiotic pills.

---

4. Sleep more and decrease your stress.
5. Don't be afraid to get a little dirty!

❧

On the flip side, having a healthy gut flora can prevent some of the damage that comes from chronic exposure to stress. Eating probiotic foods that encourage gut health and staying away from the gut wreckers will calm the brain's stress response while improving mood and even acne. Studies show improved mood and lower rates of depression, anxiety, and stress in healthy adults taking a daily probiotic supplement as compared to a placebo.

Ultimately, you will want your body to activate what we call autophagy, which is a kind of cellular cleanup that occurs when food isn't coming in. Think of it this way: When you have guests coming and going all the time at your house, you don't have a lot of time to clean up, right? Or get that light fixed that is burned out in the hallway? Your body reacts in the same way. When you have a lot of things coming in, your body won't be able to do the regular cleaning — it needs time to repair and renew. Intermittent fasting is a way to do just that, as well as a way to supercharge your gut and also aid in weight loss.

Intermittent fasting, or IF, is a super-hot topic, and study after study has shown the benefits of it. Fasting gives the body a break for a set number of hours so that your gut can repair, reset, and rest. I recommend doing some kind of intermittent fast two to three days a week (see more in the WTF plan, starting on page 183). The benefits to your gut and overall inflammation are staggering! Some people feel that intermittent fasting is key to preventing aging and inflammation and to resetting the gut.

Once you have added fiber to your diet, removed the common gut wreckers, and decreased your intake of sugar and processed gluten, you can add this as a next step. Just be careful not to do too many things at once.

Curious to learn more about IF? That's good, because that is what the next chapter is about!

6

Circadian Fasting

(aka the Fountain of Energy No One Knows About)

Y DAD GREW UP IN PALEJ, a tiny town in Western India that did not yet have electricity. Streets would be aglow with gas lamps and homes lit by candlelight. "There's only so much you can do by candlelight. So we would go to bed two to three hours after sunset. We'd wake up soon after sunrise because the sun would stream in. There were no blackout curtains back then," my dad would often tell us as kids. He was a very quiet man and hardly talked about his childhood, so when he did, we always listened intently. He would also tell us that he and his four brothers would sometimes sleep under the stars outside on their terrace, waking to the bright morning sun.

This was how it was for humans, for thousands of years before electricity was discovered. Humans awoke with the sun and went to sleep when it was dark. It was a lovely natural rhythm we shared with nature, and a natural rhythm we still carry with us today in many ways, as our internal clocks are "set" by this circadian rhythm.

Every single organism on the planet contains a "clock" that adapts to day and night — a cycle called "circadian," from the Latin words *circa* meaning "around" and *dies* meaning "day." It is our own internal clock that regulates the sleep-wake cycle and repeats roughly every 24 hours to maximize our body's own resources. Before Thomas Edison invented the lightbulb (and Steve Jobs invented the iPhone), the sun was our only source of light (besides fire), and thus all of human behavior and activity followed that natural day-night cycle, just like my father and his family did when he was growing up.

In recent years, we've learned a lot more about our circadian rhythm and what it means for our health. For instance, we've known for a long time that this inner clock is composed of a group of neurons called the "suprachiasmatic nucleus" (which sounds awfully close to the "Supercalifragilisticexpialidocious" song in *Mary Poppins*), that it resides in the hypothalamus, and that it affects our sleep and wake cycles. But what we didn't realize until recently — and are only starting to understand — is that there are individual clocks in *every cell in every one of our organs,* and they can function even without the central circadian clock. In 2017 the Nobel Prize for Medicine went to three scientists — Jeffrey C. Hall, Michael Rosbash, and Michael W. Young — "for their discoveries of molecular mechanisms controlling the circadian rhythm."[1] By studying tiny fruit flies, they isolated a gene that controls the normal daily biological rhythm and discovered how a protein accumulates in the cell during the night and is then degraded during the day.

What this tells us is that every cell has an inner clock, independent of the one that is in our brain. Just think about all the mini-timers in our skin, muscles, GI tract, heart, liver — all working on a set time. We also now know that all our cells' mitochondria — microscopic organelles that produce energy needed to function — have a relationship with our circadian rhythm, so it makes sense that *when* we eat is just as important as *what* we eat.[2] Like every living organism, every cell in our body responds to the sun rising and setting, and it is that cycle by which we set our internal clocks.

Now, just think about how we abuse this beautiful timing by constantly changing our sleep patterns and eating schedules and exposing ourselves to unfriendly environments that mess with those inner clocks.[3] Today, the inescapable fluorescent and LED lighting that's on the digital screens of our computers, cell phones, TVs, and car dashboards messes with that natural system, disrupting the natural cycle based on day and night upon which our bodily systems rely. The industrial age also brought with it the ability to travel far into different time zones, has given us 24/7 communication and news cycles, and made it possible to work the night shift, which many people do. All these industrial "advances" have been integral in ushering us into a modern age, but there have been some unintended consequences, and we are only beginning to realize their implications on our natural cycles. And while the jury is out on just how much this disruption affects our bodies, studies indicate that it's proving to be a weighty factor in our overall health and longevity. Science is just uncovering how our circadian rhythm affects our daily energy, our weight, our gut health, our mental health, and our ability to make decisions.

While the next few years should bring mounting evidence to confirm this, we should do something about it now. Don't fret. I have a plan to fix this. The answer to getting more energy is already within you — you just need to learn to better optimize it by linking your circadian rhythm with your eating and sleep cycles. But first, let's dig into the circadian rhythm a bit more so you can understand how integral it is to our health.

HOW EXACTLY DOES THE
CIRCADIAN RHYTHM WORK?

So every cell has its own clock that runs according to the body's natural circadian rhythm. These tons of tiny circadian clocks throughout the body all set their time by direct input from neurons present in our eyes that also lead to that suprachiasmatic nucleus in the brain mentioned above. At the same time, these circadian clocks get direct input from the sun. Why is this important? Until recently, we thought the suprachiasmatic nucleus was the only way that we orchestrate the circadian rhythm, but now we know that it happens on the cellular level as well. For instance, there was one strong study where they took mice that did not have the retinal neurons and they were still able to keep on a circadian clock because of their individual circadian clocks in the tissues. Pretty cool, eh?

We are in sync if we allow this natural rhythm to do its job — that is, we are active and productive during the day, and then we rest at night so our body can focus on repair.

But here is the problem: modern living is disrupting our master clock, and the clocks in every cell, so rather than running smoothly and on time, our bodies are out of sync and running on empty. If we stay up late, check Instagram at 2 a.m., or get up for a midnight snack, we sabotage that natural cycle of nightly rest and repair. Imagine trying to do several hours' worth of work in one hour (remember that analogy of always entertaining guests?). Stressful, and nearly impossible, right? Something will most likely go wrong. This is what the body tries to do, though, when we mess with our biological clock and are not giving it the right amount of sleep. When our body doesn't have the time to repair itself, it doesn't get done. The body has to triage the next day's activities but can't make up for it. Repairs that are not checked off the to-do list lead to fatigue and lack of energy and, in the long term, disease.

The Shift Worker

Kate, at 38, was a dedicated nurse at a prenatal unit at the local hospital. But her dedication was catching up to her — long hours (12-hour shifts three times a week) and a stressful environment were causing fatigue and constipation.

"I love my work and my babies. But the hours are crazy, and I think it is really affecting my energy levels. Is there anything I can do?" she asked me, clearly frustrated.

There are millions of people who work night shifts or off-hours, and while their dedication to their work is integral to keeping society going — whether it's a cop on a beat, or an emergency responder constantly at the ready, or a subway conductor managing the maze of tunnels — they are all endangering their own health. According to 2004 data from the Bureau of Labor Statistics, nearly 15 million Americans work full-time on evening shifts, night shifts, rotating shifts, or other employer-arranged irregular schedules. According to the Sleep Foundation, roughly 15 percent of full-time wage and salary workers in the US work on shifts outside the traditional daytime schedule. But as noble as their jobs are and no matter how many times they may have saved someone else's life with their work, they may be killing themselves slowly because of the regular disruption to their circadian rhythm.

Getting out of sync with your circadian rhythm triggers a host of problems (which non-shift workers who suffer from insomnia may also experience):

- During sleep, we produce human growth hormone (HGH), which is then released through the body to help it repair itself while we get our zzz's. When we sleep less, not enough growth hormone is produced to help our body repair itself.
- When we eat late at night, our stomach works to digest food instead of putting energy into repairing itself. This could lead to improper digestion (hello, acid reflux and indigestion) and, in the long term, diseases of the gut.
- A tired brain "tricks" us into thinking we're hungrier than we are by misreading how much energy is needed for the day.[4] We'll eat more and make poor food choices because the decision-making part of the brain is not working at full capacity. (Think about the last time you were tired: you kept reaching for chips and cookies, right? And you may keep eating to think it will make you feel better and more awake. This is that poor decision-making at its best.)
- If you eat late at night, your body is forced to produce insulin to address the influx of food, which will also disrupt your gut balance.[5]

More important, compelling studies show that intense work schedules have really bad health outcomes when it comes to cancer and shortened longevity. So much so that the World Health Organization has recently listed shift work as a likely carcinogen.[6]

While pointing out these dangerous effects is of no comfort to those who have to continue to work such hours, it is important to know and take steps to mitigate the worst effects. (One key strategy is to eat during daylight hours and sleep as much in nighttime hours as physically possible.)

Modern Times Are Killing Us

Innovation has brought modern-day conveniences that can have a huge effect on our circadian rhythm beyond shift work. Look around you—maybe you are reading this book on your Kindle or iPad. Is your smartphone next to you on your lap or tabletop? Are you reading this under a lamp? Maybe you'll get hungry and go to the refrigerator to get a snack—look at that, a light turns on as you open the door.

We are bombarded with blue light that is predominantly used in digital technology. In our retinas, we have a protein called melanopsin that plays an important role in both "setting" that master circadian clock in our brain and in the release of melatonin, and this protein is negatively affected by the spectrum of blue light because, unlike red or green light or even the yellowish-white light used in lightbulbs, blue light signals your brain to stay awake and affects the production of our sleep hormone, melatonin.[7]

In fact, one of the biggest upsets in our circadian rhythm is with our melatonin. Normally produced at night to help us feel tired so we can go into repair mode, melatonin gets shut down or delays production when exposed to blue light. Computers, tablets, and phones with blue-light screens ruin our sleep, yes, but the health effects disrupting your circadian rhythm go far beyond shut-eye. One hour of blue light delays melatonin production for three hours and reduces peak melatonin by 50 percent.[8]

Working in artificial light at night may also lower melatonin levels; and melatonin has been known to suppress tumor development, raising the stakes in developing cancer. And you don't have to be a shift worker to have this wreak havoc on your system — jet lag or too much blue or artificial light (you still reading on your Kindle?) could be damaging the very cells that make our bodies function.

We are only just beginning to understand what the impact of blue light can be on our overall health, but we do understand that artificial light can be detected by the body whether you're directly looking at light or not, even if you're just sitting in a room with a lamp on. Your retinas and other cells in your body can sense that light in the room, which sets off a chain of reactions (or, in some cases, suppresses reactions) that keep you up and give your repair guys the night off. Blue light is killing us slowly, plain and simple.

We also know that the rushed frenzy of modern life affects how much sleep we get, and this has major repercussions as well. Getting only six hours of sleep is almost as bad as getting none at all, and it's proven that sleep loss impacts your cognition, your immune system, your energy, your gut health, even your DNA. Another eye-opening stat: men who slept five hours or less had testosterone levels of men six to ten years their senior. (This study didn't examine women, but it's likely this hormonal detriment happens across genders.)

It's clear that a combination of blue light, disruptive sleep patterns, travel to different time zones, and not getting the right amount of sleep can be a recipe for disaster.

WHAT CAN WE DO?

Now that I scared you seven ways from Sunday about how our modern times are killing us (not that we had enough to worry about!), let me put you at ease. There are simple changes that can help you recalibrate your system:

- First, go to bed and get up at the same time every day. This will help with the steady production of melatonin.
- Second, have that sleep be restful, sleeping 7–9 hours most nights.

- Third, limit exposure to blue light in the evening as much as you can (such as watching TV, staring at your phone, or walking around in a brightly lit grocery store).
- Fourth (saving the best for last), follow my circadian fasting program. As we now know, the gut is key to our overall health, but we can't achieve a healthy gut without being mindful of our circadian rhythm.

WTF IS CIRCADIAN FASTING?

The old saying "eat after six, forever on your hips!" may not be just a silly old wives' tale after all. Giving our bodies a rest from food can be very beneficial to our overall health, and "gut rest" is exactly that — you are giving your gut a much-needed rest. This means you stop eating 2–3 hours before bed and fast until late in the morning. There have been a plethora of studies that show that eating in this window (late morning to early evening/late afternoon) is super beneficial to our insulin levels and sleep. And, as we know, good sleep helps the body reboot and repair itself. For example, studies show that for every 3-hour increase in nighttime fasting, there was a 4 percent reduction in glucose. This means that if we stop eating 3 hours before bed, we'll be rewarded over the long term with less diabetes, heart disease, and obesity. (Maybe my grandmother was omniscient, as she always told me not to eat 3 hours before bedtime.)

Intermittent fasting has been a hot diet buzzword for a few years now — it was the most googled diet in 2019![9] — and for good reason: the program is great for our health. There is a ton of data about how giving your body a break from food is enormously beneficial to your waistline and well-being. Studies have shown that IF makes us less insulin resistant and gives us far more energy, better cognition and memory, and increased production of neurotrophic growth factor, a protein that promotes neuron growth and protection.[10] There have been studies on different groups showing some cardiovascular, cognitive, blood sugar, and weight loss benefits on IF. Fasting intermittently can also prime your cells so they can better handle stressful insults. One study says that a break from eating jolts cells into a minor stressful state, making them more capable of later fending off other types of stress — like the kind that can lead to disease. The limitation of these studies is they tended to be small and short term; there haven't been enough human studies to really give us all the details of how often and how long fasts should be for optimum benefit. But exciting research continues to come out to confirm IF's possibilities, and in December 2019 the *New England Journal of Medicine* reviewed multiple studies on the health effects of IF confirming those results, and it went on to say that fasting then feeding can create a "cascade of changes including enhanced DNA repair, mitochondria biogenesis, decreased inflammation."[11] Let's take a deeper dive into what exactly all this means.

Autophagy

One of the goals for any fasting program is to ramp up the body's autophagy (which literally translates into "self-eating"), which, if you remember from page 120, is the body's way of self-cleaning and self-regeneration. Autophagy is always happening at a low level. The point is to accelerate it. We don't have a way to really measure autophagy — it happens at different times for different people — but it seems like ketosis, a metabolic state that uses fat for fuel instead of glucose, sets it off. For many people, ketosis and autophagy start at the 16-hour point (fasted workouts can help you get into autophagy sooner). In this state, our bodies are able to clean out damaged cells so we can regenerate newer, healthier cells, and this can't happen unless you take away your body's food resources. This shift in calorie sources causes your body to go into ketosis.

This low glucagon level is what initiates autophagy. Like a light dimmer, it turns up the survival repairing mode of autophagy. So deep is this cleaning that if you look at a cell that has undergone autophagy, you cannot tell the difference between that cell and a younger cell. It is like anti-aging treatment — without needles! We are not sure when that happens, but depending on your protein and sugar reserves, real autophagy can really ramp up at the 14-, 16-, 18-, and definitely at the 24-hour mark.

While the longer you can hold off from eating the better (within reason, of course), we know there are great benefits with fasting even if autophagy is not technically reached. Intermittent fasting sets off what the *New England Journal of Medicine* article calls "metabolic switching" — going back and forth between using glucose (when not fasting) and using fatty acids (when fasting) as a source of energy. This seems to be the magic of intermittent fasting, which, along with the natural caloric restriction that comes with skipping a meal (or two), kicks off protective mechanisms and strengthens so many of our cellular processes.[12]

Our bodies appear to adapt to this on-off switch by bolstering mitochondrial function (how energy is made), stress resistance, and antioxidant defenses while in the fasting phase or autophagy state; in other words, when going from fasting to feeding, the body can repair and get stronger than it was before. When we are fasting, glucose levels decrease as ketones go up, and cells continue to grow and repair. As the *New England Journal of Medicine* article explains, the long-term benefits of IF, particularly when coupled with regular exercise, include improvements in mental and physical functionality and gut microbiota, weight loss, a decrease in inflammation, and help in staving off disease.[13] Simply put, we get metabolically "stronger" every time we fast. Our DNA repair is better, our mitochondrial production (i.e., making energy) is more robust, our autophagy state is heightened, while inflammation is mitigated. This adaptive response to fasting is seen in all species, not just humans. But most people in the modern world don't benefit because they never go into a fasting state!

Fasting Can Reduce Cancer

The same *New England Journal of Medicine* article documents
a number of clinical trials, while still in the testing phases,
that show promising cancer-reducing effects of intermittent
fasting. One followed patients with an aggressive form of
brain cancer (glioblastoma) and showed that IF suppressed
tumor growth and improved survival rates. Promising
studies have also shown how intermittent fasting reduces
the signaling in insulin-like growth hormone factor 1 (IGF-1)
and growth hormone that can cause cancer growth. Another
indicated notable increases in activity of certain transcription
factors that are protective in cancer growth pathways, offering
promising opportunities in cancer treatment.[14] There was also
a 2016 study done on a group of women who had a history
of breast cancer; it followed them over time as they fasted
an average of 13.5 hours a night. Amazingly, they found a 36
percent reduction in breast cancer recurrence.[15]

I've seen these results firsthand with myself and in my practice.
My patient Julia is a perfect case study. A busy musician, she was always on a plane, a train, or in a car traveling for her gigs. Because of
her constant on-the-go lifestyle, she had suffered from weight gain,
lethargy, and high blood pressure. Fed up, she came to see me.

"I have heard so much about intermittent fasting and want to try
it, but I am so confused which fast is best. There are just so many out
there!" she said to me as she sat in my office one day.

"I have found certain types of fasting to be pretty stressful on the
body, and for a busy person like yourself, you don't need to be so extreme. Let's talk about your daily food intake and try to make it doable for *you*," I said. We then discussed what would fit her lifestyle,
and we decided that 12 hours of fasting daily was a good start for her
while she worked on getting her stress levels under control (this is
key when you are trying to fast and balance hormones). In addition,

she decided to cut out sugar completely from her diet except for fruit and other naturally occurring sugars. She also started doing nature walks daily.

After two weeks of a cleaner diet, 12-hour fasting, and daily walks, she felt remarkably better. Kate, the shift worker, also felt like a new person after I had given her an individualized IF plan that would work best according to her schedule.

Religious Fasting

To date, modern cultures haven't really taken advantage of these fasting mechanisms at all.[16] Yet we have seen fasting used as part of many older religious or spiritual practices: Islam, Christianity, Judaism, and Buddhism all have certain fasting rituals, which is interesting to note considering the new science that speaks to the health benefits of fasting. In some cases, these religious practices have aided in better understanding the potential health benefits of fasting. There have been studies, for instance, on Muslims participating in their monthlong Ramadan — a religious holiday that calls for people to fast from food and water from dawn until sunset — that indicate IF improves the immune system and heart health and lowers diabetes risk.[17]

There are a few popular IF diets out there. Most of you probably have heard of the 16/8 fast, one of the more popular fasting programs, which calls for taking a break from eating for 16 hours — typically from 8 p.m. to noon the next day — allowing yourself only water or black coffee and sometimes a very small snack depending on the protocol followed. This type of fasting is immensely popular, but it's not what I would recommend to start. A typical American eats during a 15-hour window, so I suggest starting to slow that down with a 12-hour fast — typically from 7 p.m. to 7 a.m., which has the added benefit of timing the fast with our internal clocks. I call this circadian fasting. Then people can graduate and do longer fasts as they acclimate to the 12-hour fasting, going up to a 14-hour or even an 18-hour fast. Anything longer than 24 hours is considered a prolonged fast.

---

4 Mistakes Made While Intermittent Fasting

Look, it is easy to make rookie mistakes on this program— I certainly did! And there are times that cravings will come into play. Here are a few tips on what to avoid and to keep yourself on track:

1. People go too long, too hard. Since you are literally starving your body, if your body is not used to it, IF will result in fatigue and cravings, and can negatively affect your hormones.
2. People don't decrease their sugar intake. If you fast and then eat too much sugar during the eating window, your body will start on a sugar-and-carb roller coaster that will negatively affect how it functions, giving you a case of the jitters along with hunger pangs and cravings.
3. People give in to cravings while fasting and go overboard and eat too much. If you are in a fasting window, try my 40-calorie snacks (page 197) to stave off those pangs.
4. People don't personalize the fast, neglecting to take into account individual health needs, such as chronic issues, pregnancy, gender, and age.

INTERMITTENT FASTING IS GOOD, BUT CIRCADIAN FASTING IS BETTER!

In the last chapter, we talked about how important gut health is, but I left out one important factor: good gut bacteria are also in sync with your body's circadian biology, which makes them more active or less active depending on the time of day. So guess what, that simpatico relationship will be affected if you eat in the middle of the night or even stay up late catching up on the latest season of Netflix's *Indian Matchmaking*. As we have seen with shift workers, when you mess with your natural eating cycle, the body will produce drowsy-making chemicals when you are on the job at night, and stimulating chemicals during the day, pushing you to be awake when you're trying to sleep.

So while I just gave you a lot of great information on how intermittent fasting or gut rest is so good for our bodies, many people are still missing a HUGE piece of the puzzle: how important circadian rhythm is to our gut and how it can play into scheduling IF to optimize fasting for the most beneficial results.

Different Types of Fasting and Time-Restricted Eating

Fasting has been a practice throughout human evolution, often out of necessity. Ancestral hunter-gatherers didn't have the luxury of having food literally at their fingertips 24 hours a day. They were dependent on hunting and foraging for their food — sometimes going for long periods of time without eating. So our bodies are actually designed for periods without food, and chances are that our ancestors weren't eating three organized meals each day or grazing on snacks all afternoon.

Times have changed, but lately there has been a rise in the popularity of diets that recognize the benefits of scheduled fasting. I'm talking about a fasting period of 12–24 hours daily — or for a few days a week — where nothing but water and low- or no-calorie beverages are consumed. Just as you and I need sleep to reset and revitalize, so do our digestive tract and organs. IF has many approaches, but all fall within two categories: alternate-day fasting and restricted eating windows. Alternate-day fasting has you eating more on some days than others, when you eat practically nothing. Restricted eating is just limiting the time in which you eat during the day. Here are some of the more popular IF methods:

- 5:2 (or the Fast Diet): The popular UK diet has you eat a regular diet five days a week and limit calories to 500 per day for two days each week.
- Warrior Diet or One Meal a Day (OMAD): Fast for 20 hours and then eat one large (healthy) meal.
- The 16/8 method: Also called the Leangains protocol, it involves skipping breakfast and restricting your daily eating period to 8 hours, such as 1–9 p.m. Then you fast for 16 hours in between.
- Eat Stop Eat: This involves fasting for 24 hours, once or twice a week, by not eating from dinner one day until dinner the next day.

One more thing: While fasting concentrates on restricting eating times, there is also calorie restriction (CR), which restricts daily food intake — usually about 25–50 percent less than the average person's intake. The science is clear that CR is a great strategy for extending a healthy life span. And when you think about it, IF is a type of CR. But IF looks as though it may be more beneficial than CR: a recent study tested a group who followed a 25 percent calorie-reduction diet against a 5:2 fasting group; while both groups lost the same amount of weight, the fasting group had greater insulin sensitivity and a larger reduction in waist circumference.[18]

The time period in which we fast needs to be taken into account, not just the total number of hours of fasting. If you think about it, there is an optimal hour we should stop eating. But most people disregard that. You can't be doing everything all the time. There have been countless studies that have shown that fasting is good for our bodies, but for fasting to truly "multitask," it should work in tandem with your own circadian rhythm. This means beginning the fasting window earlier in the day and ending it earlier. For example, in my plan, you would eat your meals between 9 a.m. and 6 p.m. or 8 a.m. and 8 p.m.

The number one no-no is eating late into the evening, which has a huge disruptive effect on our cells. When you eat late at night, your cells are not optimized to expect glucose at that time. If you cause cortisol to spike in the middle of the night because you're super stressed or are digesting food, your body can't do the necessary repairs during its downtime because it is too busy making that cortisol. If you do things according to your natural circadian rhythm, you'll achieve better hormonal balance and long-term health.

Need more proof that this works? Circadian rhythm expert Dr. Satchin Panda conducted a study where he took mice from the same mother, identical in age and gender, and fed one group an around-the-clock high-fat/high-sucrose diet, and the other group the same diet but with a limited 8-hour eating window. Both groups ate the same number of calories, with 60 percent from fat, 20 percent from sucrose, and the rest from protein. After 18 weeks, the mice who followed the 8-hour eating window weighed 28 percent less on average. To verify these findings, Dr. Panda repeated this experiment three times, with similar results. The mice in the fasting group also showed increased endurance (thought to be a benefit from the presence of ketone in the blood).

Need more proof? I have promoted the circadian fasting plan to many of my patients, most of whom have marveled at their transformations. Madeline, for example, was experiencing fatigue and low energy throughout the day, and she also felt irritable at her job. As a cardiology physician assistant, that kind of impatience is just not an option. I had her start out doing intermittent fasting three days a week (on days she wasn't working out). She would start eating no earlier than 8 a.m. and have to be done eating by 8 p.m.; the next day, she could have a black coffee in the morning but would wait to eat lunch at noon. I also had Madeline try to get to bed by 9 or 9:30 p.m. to get a full eight hours of sleep.

After a few months, she came back into my office for a checkup.

"So, how did it go?" I asked, excited to hear her thoughts.

"Dr. Shah! Crazy good! Number one, I didn't realize how much sleep I really needed until I went to bed so early. I can't tell you how the intermittent fasting has made a huge difference already. I am no longer eating willy-nilly whenever I want; the structure really works for me. And the best part, I am no longer losing my patience at work, and my energy hangs around all day. I am like a new person!"

Now that is what I love to hear. Happy patients make me happy.

Another satisfied customer is closer to home — my husband, Akshay. A few years ago he, at 39, was at the pinnacle of his career, but he was feeling extra tired. Part of it was the middle-aged doldrums, for sure, but he just didn't feel like his normal energized self. Based on my encouragement, he started circadian fasting and quickly saw his mental acuity improve, and he felt like he had a better outlook on life. He also lost weight. It's been three years of transformation: he's 40 pounds lighter, his mood is better, and his energy has surged. "Even as a board-certified physician, I never fully understood the link between my gut health and my energy levels until I started doing this," he marveled to me. Do you know what is super cool? While this helped him connect to himself better mentally and spiritually, it also helped us connect better as a couple; with a clearer headspace, he was more attuned to my feelings and needs. Not a bad side effect!

What Chronotype Are You?

Are you a night owl or an early bird? Most people insist that they are one or the other, but night owls become that way either by drinking coffee too late in the day, or by watching TV, using their e-book readers, scrolling through their smartphone, or having any kind of light that disrupts their sleep and leaves them more susceptible to health problems. Most people are, in fact, very similar in their circadian rhythms — it's the external stimuli that make them *think* they are night owls. That said, those who do like stay up late and sleep later could adjust their eating window to later in the day to match their schedule.

Our Circadian Rhythm Ages, Too

For most of our lives, our circadian rhythm is steady as she goes. But as we age, our CR can begin to shift. And we see it affect our sleep in terms of timing, quality, and duration. Older adults sleep less, as well as going to bed and waking up earlier than they used to. (That's why early bird specials are so popular, I guess!) Their cognitive function also may be worse at nighttime.[19]

HOW TO INCORPORATE CIRCADIAN FASTING IN YOUR LIFE

We'll get into the details of the plan later in the book, but I want to give you a bird's-eye view of how circadian fasting works, and how better eating habits can optimize your body's natural biological clock. First things first, intermittent fasting is different for men than it is for women.

Women Fast Differently

If you are a woman reading this book, chances are you've experienced the diet roller coaster at least once — if not dozens of times — in your life, just as I had. At first, intermittent fasting seemed to be another "lose weight fast" fad, so I quit. That was before I realized that women need to fast differently.

Women are very sensitive to starvation and to stress on our bodies because our bodies are wired to detect starvation and nutrition deficiencies. Able to carry children, women's bodies are particularly tuned into the potential nutritional needs of pregnancy and nursing (this is all an evolutionary hypothesis). Many women try intermittent fasting and will see that their periods are off, or they miss their period, or they're having other issues with their cycle. That's a sign that IF is too stressful for your body. I tell my patients that if there's a change in your cycle, that's a feedback signal from your body that the fast you are doing is too aggressive for you or fasting is not for you at all.

When I first tried IF, I did what a lot of people do: I jumped right into it. I wanted to be an A+ overachiever student, and because I started too aggressively, I failed desperately. By day three, I was already fatigued and felt like my cravings were markedly increased. I wasn't sleeping well and had trouble exercising. And I was pushing through to the point where I was not functioning. So after about a week of this, I quit and said, "There's something off here."

What I didn't realize back then is that women experience intermittent fasting quite differently than men. It's sometimes trickier for women to get results. The physiological and weight benefits are still possible, but sometimes require a different approach.

In fact, if not done right, IF may cause a hormonal imbalance in women because we are extremely sensitive to signals of starvation.[20] If the body senses starvation, it will kick up the production of hunger hormones. Therefore, when you break the fast, you may experience insatiable hunger. It's our body's way of protecting a potential fetus (even when we're not pregnant). Many of us driven, busy women tend to not notice those hunger cues. Or even worse, we purposely ignore them, then fail and binge later, but follow that up with undereating and starvation again. Guess what? All that can halt ovulation. Remember those GnRH pulses we discussed in chapter 1? Those pulses in women seem to be very sensitive to stressors like intermittent fasting.

All that being said, I think that most people, even those of reproductive age, will do fine with gentle fasting, as long as when you eat, you do it healthfully. There are some animal studies that have shown that aggressive extended fasting (nearly 48 hours) halted the menstrual cycle in female rats after two weeks and their ovaries shrunk, and male rats ended up with lower testosterone production.[21] But there aren't any human studies that have looked at fasting for women specifically, so we are relying on tests that have been done on mice that were on a very aggressive fasting schedule — not the best proxy for humans.

What I have found with my own fasting and my own patients' is that while an extended form of fasting can sometimes throw off a woman's hormonal balance and cause fertility problems, the benefits seem to greatly outweigh the unconfirmed side effects. So my advice for women is to go really low and slow and let the body and hormones acclimate. The best way to do that is what I call "crescendo" intermittent fasting because you're gradually working your body until you find the fasting approach that is sustainable for you.

Fasting on nonconsecutive days and having "eating windows" can help you achieve the benefits of IF without the hormonal downswing. I suggest starting with a 12- to 16-hour fast three days a week (but not three days in a row). On those three days, you should focus on healthy eating during a restricted window — say, from 10:00 a.m. to 7:00 p.m. Typically, you can achieve this by just delaying breakfast. Make sure to do a shorter training session on fast days. It should be "shorter" for you, so for me that means doing HIIT or something less intense like yoga.

- Eat normally on your high-cardio days (that means one or more intense hours of running, biking, metabolic conditioning, interval training, etc.). This can be modified once you are more experienced at fasting.
- Drink plenty of water. Tea and coffee are okay, too.

After you get comfortable with this (after two to three weeks), feel free to fast more often and add challenges like fasting for longer on weekends and for less time on weekdays.

Keep in mind that this might not work for everyone, but this plan has worked for many women: I have put hundreds of women on a circadian fasting plan with phenomenal results. I also think circadian fasting is really doable for busy people, because it is so darn easy to remember. I have actually had several patients comment on how they like making the gut rest a game ("Let's see, can I do a 16-hour fast today?"), which can be so motivating. While the jury is out on what is the optimum fasting time frame, the longer you can go, ideally up to 16 hours, the more benefit you'll see. But that type of fasting is not sustainable (that is why some of these 16/8 fasting diets are just fads), which is why I don't recommend a 16-hour fast every day for most people. And just be careful that you don't go too long without eating; that will sabotage your efforts altogether. Most people can benefit from just 12 hours.

That Other Cycle and Circadian Fasting

Women have a unique hormonal cycle, and when electing to do this type of fasting, they need to take this into consideration. Because of our hormonal fluctuation, I like to suggest to my patients that during the first half of their cycle (days 0–14), when your hormones are low and rising (follicular phase) and estrogen is relatively dominant, you can be aggressive with IF. You could do a 16-hour fast 2–3 times a week, work out harder, and eat more healthy carbs. During the second half (days 15–28, the luteal phase), when hormone levels rise then drop (and energy naturally dips) and progesterone is relatively dominant, ease up on fasting as well as working out, and curb your carb intake. If you find yourself experiencing any changes to your cycle while doing an intermittent fast, stop immediately. Assuming your symptoms normalize after a couple of weeks, I suggest trying a more modified version of IF such as a 12-hours-only circadian fast. (We'll go more into this in chapter 8.)

Avoiding food between the hours of 8 p.m. to 8 a.m. or 7 p.m. to 7 a.m. is a good baseline. You can also experience great benefits with a 14-hour period, where you would eat from 10 a.m. to 8 p.m. These 12- or 14-hour fasts may be less trendy, but if we're going for the long haul and creating a new lifestyle versus trying a crash diet, this time frame is much more attainable and manageable. Once you're comfortable with the 12-hour fast, you can work up to fasting 16 hours in a stretch two to three times a week, from 8 p.m. to noon the next day.

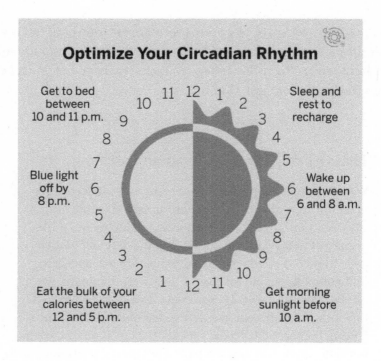

Optimize Your Circadian Rhythm

Get to bed between 10 and 11 p.m.

Sleep and rest to recharge

Blue light off by 8 p.m.

Wake up between 6 and 8 a.m.

Eat the bulk of your calories between 12 and 5 p.m.

Get morning sunlight before 10 a.m.

I get it — everyone is busy with a career, a social life, and a family. An 8 a.m.–8 p.m. eating schedule may work for one woman but may not work for the next. If these hours don't fit your schedule, shift to what does work for you, keeping three things constant: First, the fasting window needs to be 12 hours. Second, this window should be as close to the circadian clock as possible. And third, stop eating three hours before you go to sleep. If you have a big party or event that will pose a challenge to the eating window, that is why I made a rest day — work that party into your fasting schedule so you can have that day fall on your rest day and enjoy yourself!

When you are fasting, always check in with yourself that you are on the right path with these surefire signs: How's your sleep? How's your energy? How are your cravings and hunger? How are your monthly cycles? Are you feeling better than you have in the past? Or worse? Monitoring yourself is a way to gauge where to go from there, either taking it to the next level or tweaking your hours to make the fast work for you.

Can IF Be a Slippery Slope for Those with Eating Disorders?

Anorexia nervosa is a serious and potentially life-threatening psychological disorder characterized as an intense fear of gaining weight. Someone with anorexia becomes severely underweight by restricting the number of calories and the types of food they eat — literally starving themselves — and ignoring their body's hunger and nutritional needs. Someone susceptible may see IF as a convenient package to indulge their obsession, but when IF is done right, satiety and nutrition are not an issue, and IF can have enormous health benefits. It is well known that women are more vulnerable to eating disorders, and so if you are someone who has a history of food issues (including bingeing and orthorexia), you probably should not do intermittent fasting, at least on your own. Do it with a friend or spouse to keep you on the right track or, better yet, consult with a medical professional who knows your condition and can provide some guidelines for you.

WHEN NOT TO FAST

And, finally, fasting isn't for everyone. We have talked about how fasting can be a challenge for women if they go in too strong. And for women who are pregnant or breastfeeding or trying to become pregnant, I suggest not partaking in intermittent fasting as there hasn't been a whole lot of research on the effects of IF on pregnancy. Play it safe. The same goes if you have a chronic condition, such as heart disease or diabetes. Also consult your doctor if you're taking any medications before trying this or any kind of fasting program.

Our bodies are made perfectly — and they are designed to repair and restore themselves at night. Let's harness this power to energize ourselves and improve our chances to live a longer, healthier life. Once you understand how circadian fasting works, you'll see how crucial it is to our health and longevity. That natural cycle is key to maintaining your body's ability to repair itself, keeping your energy levels in tip-top shape, and staving off disease. If you are tired, it may be because you are not optimizing your body's own repair system. Don't fight the system. Work with the system with time-restricted eating. Lo and behold, you will feel better and more energized in no time!

INTERMITTENT FASTING CHEAT SHEET

1. The *best type* of intermittent fasting for a busy person, in my opinion, is circadian fasting, which means eating for an 8- to 10-hour window during the day. If you are new to IF, then start slow, fasting for 12 hours and eating for 12 hours. *There are no hard rules, except that you need to respect and listen to your body.*
2. Cycle your fast. If I fast for 12 hours one day, then I switch it to 14 or 16 hours the next. I find that it's kinder to my hormones and less stressful.
3. Try to cluster most of your calories from 12 p.m. to 5 p.m. Try not to eat within 3 hours of bedtime, and do not overeat during your eating window. Plan your meals and eating times in advance. A good guide is to break your fast with something small between 8 and 10 a.m., with lunch at 12 and then dinner between 3 and 6, if your schedule allows.
4. Nutrient-dense foods are best: nuts, seeds, fruits (berries), vegetables, lean protein (sprouted tofu), whole grains, beans. Focus on eating high-fiber, unprocessed, whole foods. Avoid meat as much as possible, especially red meat, sugar, trans fats, and refined starches.
5. If you get hungry during your fasting period, try to curb your hunger with water or non-caloric drinks (such as coffee and

tea). If your hunger does not dissipate, then eat something that is sugar-free and is 40 calories or less, such as a spoonful of peanut butter, a thin slice of avocado, or a handful of nuts.

6. Fasted workouts, where you work out at the end of the fasting period, will give you the best chance to get the full metabolic benefits of fasting, such as metabolic switching. It also ramps up the autophagy mode, which is so regenerating. Time a meal to follow a moderate to aggressive workout. (Some people cannot exercise on an empty stomach, so if that is the case, eat first, then exercise.)

7. Stay hydrated while fasting. Drink 2.25–2.75 litres of water per day.

8. Constantly check in with your body. If your answer to any of these questions is concerning, stop your fast and check in with your doctor: *Is your energy stable? Are your periods regular, or are you missing or having irregular periods? How are your cravings and hunger? How are you sleeping?*

9. Intermittent fasting is not a "lose weight quick" scheme. You need to have the right mindset for IF. Make sure you have clear and concise objectives for your fasting program.

10. Get plenty of rest. Sleep a minimum of 7 hours per night (if not more). Also, a 20-minute catnap during the day can do wonders for your body. If you can squeeze in a quick nap, take advantage and recharge.

7

All Together Now

JOAN IS PROBABLY LIKE MANY of you. She subscribes to umpteen magazines (that may or may not pile up on her coffee table) and follows health bloggers and Instagrammers, trying to keep up with the latest on health news. Always on the lookout for the next new diet, she was careful about what she ate, but she had been on as many diets as there are months in a year, all touting to regain the energy of her youth, but nothing really worked in the long term. She was still feeling tired, but hoping to find *something* that would bring her energy back, she came to me.

"Dr. Shah, I am just *so* confused with the mountain of information out there — so much of it is contradictory. One day gluten is out; the next day it is back in. Keto was so hot for a while, but now I am reading it isn't good for you in the long term . . . Trying to figure out what to eat is exhausting. Every day there seems to be a new study that debunks yesterday's study, a new diet that outdoes last week's diet. How can we keep up?"

We can't. But I am here to say we don't have to.

Within these pages, I have shown you that our gut, immune system, and hormones are all connected: your brain is connected to your hormones, which are connected to your gut, which is connected to your immune system, and it loops back around on that heavily trafficked interconnected highway. So now that you know about this connection, *how can you optimize it?* That's the goal, right? You know the old saying that the way to a man's heart is through his stomach? Well, we can steal from this a bit and say that the way to a healthy body is through your gut. I believe by eating right and keeping your gut flora balanced and healthy, you can maintain that important balance in the energy trifecta.

And because everything is connected, we need to have our diet dialed into that connection. So many people have been eating for either gut health or eating for hormone health or for inflammation. Western medicine and the media would still have you believe that we need to treat every system separately. But I believe that to maximize our health and energy, we need a diet plan that works for the entire energy trifecta. Because as you now have read, if you have cortisol imbalance, you probably have immune issues and gut issues as well — our diet needs to be multifaceted and timed to work with the entire system. If we can modify our diet to work for the energy trifecta, a whole lot of healing can happen: we boost our immune system, promote gut health, and our energy levels will shoot up.

WHAT MOVES THE NEEDLE ON YOUR ENERGY LEVELS?

First and foremost, I am a big promoter of a good diet for energy. For me and what I have seen in my patients, the right foods move the needle the most. Nearly as important is our sleep, exercise, and controlling stress.

NOM NOM NOM: WHAT TO EAT

There are a few major factors that keep that energy trifecta in good working order, but the biggest needle mover? *Food*. What you put in your mouth is going to be the most important predictor of your energy levels and overall health.

My food suggestions for gaining that energy trifecta are very close to those foods recommended in the Mediterranean diet, not coincidentally as it has proven to lower inflammation, although I modify it to fit our modern needs. The Mediterranean diet, and the diet I recommend in the WTF plan, is largely plant-based, with a high intake of healthy fats, fiber, and natural sugars from olive oil, fruit, nuts, and vegetables. It also calls for little (or no) dairy products, meat, or sweets; and wine in moderation.

Many studies, including one in the *New England Journal of Medicine,* support this. Mediterranean-style diets have been shown over and over again to be preventative for heart disease. In addition to that, research shows that plant-based diets are cost-effective, low-risk interventions that may lower body mass index, blood pressure, blood sugar, and cholesterol levels.

Mediterranean-style diets may also reduce the number of medications needed to treat chronic diseases and lower heart disease mortality rates. Also, the Adventist Health Studies — a long-term research project that studies the lifestyles of Seventh-day Adventists, who are believed to be healthier and live longer due to their diet and healthy habits — found that vegetarians have approximately half the risk of developing diabetes as non-vegetarians.[1] Likewise, the Dietary Guidelines Advisory Committee, an advisory board within the federal government, found that plant-based diets were associated with a reduced risk of cardiovascular disease and mortality compared with non-plant-based diets. (Again, meat and fish are fine as long as 90 percent of your diet is plant-based.) Pretty impressive findings, right? Here are a few must-haves to include in your diet.

The Essentials

Fiber, the Silent Hero

If there is one thing I have learned from all my research, it's that you need fiber to keep the gut in good working order. Fiber may not be the sexiest thing around — it's mostly known as a supplement for helping your bowels to, uh, move — but I'd love to change our conception of fiber. American culture has treated protein like a rock star, whereas fiber is treated like a roadie. When I talk about fiber to my clients, they often mistakenly ask, "What brand?" I am not talking about adding some powder to your drink. I am talking about fiber that comes from real food. And the best source of fiber is from plants: think broccoli and bottoms of asparagus, kale stems, sweet potatoes, ginger, leeks, legumes, beans. A 2019 review of 250 studies confirmed that eating lots of fiber from natural sources can decrease heart disease, lower cholesterol levels, and reduce cancer morbidity.[2] Eat to good health, as they say!

Two Types of Fiber

Not all fiber is the same — and the differences can get more complicated than we need to get into here — but let's look at the two main types:

Soluble fiber dissolves in water and turns into a gel-like substance during digestion, which helps slow down the process. Black beans, broccoli, apples, avocado, and sweet potatoes are all great sources for this kind of fiber.

Insoluble fiber is fiber that does not break down in the digestive system, but works as an aid to help move food through our stomach and intestines. It's like a Hoover for your digestive system. Cauliflower, green beans, whole-wheat flour and bran, and nuts are all good forms of insoluble fiber.

Prebiotic fiber. Prebiotic fiber has taken a back seat to its more famous cousin, probiotics, which are live bacteria found in yogurt and other fermented foods. Prebiotic fiber — abundantly found in asparagus, chicory root, leeks, onions, and garlic, but you really can't go wrong with any vegetable — encourages the growth of the good bacteria already in the gut. Think of it as a fertilizer for the good gut bacteria. Probiotics are good, but prebiotics are better because they prime the gut for the healthy bacteria of probiotics.

Eat your vegetables. Because of the decreased nutritional value and loss of diversity in grains, they should be a smaller part of our diet. (And those grains should be whole grains, not processed.) We need to really increase the amount of vegetables — sourcing local and organic is best — to amounts most Americans do not get: 6–8 servings a day. Why? Vegetables contain a lot of that important fiber we just discussed, as well as hundreds to thousands of phytonutrients — literally plant hormones — that have a hormone-balancing effect in the body. Vegetables (as well as fruit) also supply us with fiber that binds itself to old estrogen, thereby clearing it out of the system, leading to better overall equilibrium. This is great for both men and women who suffer from estrogen dominance.

But the biggest plus is that vegetables also supply prebiotic fibers that good bacteria feed on in the gut. You want to eat vegetables that have the prebiotic benefits, for sure, and there are also the inflammatory benefits. It's no longer just opinion or up for debate — eating more plants or a primarily plant-based diet is better for preventing and treating inflammation-based disease. And you want the plants you eat to be as diverse as possible. Growing studies show that the more variety you have in your plant intake, the more diverse (and thus healthy) bacteria in your gut. By the way, stressed plants — meaning plants that were grown in non-ideal conditions, like a period of drought or too much water — are even more fibrous. While we can't choose plants based on this factor, we know they are helpful for our digestion either way. Just another reason to eat our veggies.

Another good rule of thumb is for the lion's share of your veggies to be green. This is one of the most simple, important keys to optimal health that is glazed over in favor of supplements and diet fads. Why? Greens are the most nutrient-dense food by far: greens contain phytonutrients, phytochemicals, vitamins, and minerals not found in supplements. There are literally thousands of phytochemicals in a stalk of broccoli that are missed out on in a supplement. When our immunity is robbed of phytonutrients, our bodies are less effective in staving off inflammation. Greens also help the body fight free-radical and cell damage that can lead to cancer and other diseases. High in fiber and in antioxidants, greens help strengthen the immune system and promote healthy intestinal flora.

Need More Ammo on Why You Should Eat Your Veggies?

Here are several reasons:

- Vegetables contain phytonutrients, phytochemicals, vitamins, and minerals that are not found in supplements.
- Greens help the body fight free-radical and cell damage that can lead to cancer and other diseases, and they keep us healthy and energized.
- Vegetables are high in antioxidants.

- They strengthen the immune system.
- They promote healthy intestinal flora.
- They clear congestion.

Also, vegetables are low in calories, high in fiber, and filling: eat 1 or 2 servings of greens at each meal, and you'll be less likely to feel hungry.

ENERGY BOOSTER

Green bananas, also a good source of prebiotics, are rich in resistant starches that, when fermented by gut bacteria, produce short-chain fatty acids (SCFAs) that literally feed the good bacteria in the gut. Resistant starches — starches that resist digestion and help feed good gut bacteria, like those in green bananas — have been shown to increase satiety and decrease hunger. They also improve glucose control after eating and help colon health.

So the takeaway here? Eat five servings of prebiotic fiber every day. Don't count calories, count fiber.

We know that our ancestors from as little as a hundred years ago were eating five times the fiber that we eat today, and their gut health was much healthier. They didn't have the stomach and digestive issues we have now. And do you know why? It's because of the proliferation of processed foods in the last fifty years. Most Americans get less than 20 grams of fiber a day, and fiber is sorely needed for good gut bacteria to grow. Worse, convenient packaged foods are made up of mostly sugar, which "feeds" bad bacteria and "starves" good bacteria.

❧

It's time that fiber from whole foods gets the A-list treatment in your diet.

Tea

Okay, coffee drinkers, listen up. Our ancestors were on to something (again) in that they drank tea for hundreds of years before the coffee bean was extracted and Starbucks was born. And really, outside of the US, tea is the most frequently ingested liquid after water, much more than coffee. In Britain a "cuppa" is the answer to *everything*.

Teas have tons of benefits — they contain almighty antioxidants. And tea is one of the most anti-inflammatory foods outside of fiber. Tea is something that has consistently shown to be healing for the body. Recent studies confirm the benefits of tea, including its hormone-balancing, anti-carcinogenic, anti-bacterial, and possible prebiotic effects. Tea gives you energy, it's inexpensive, and it's effective.

The longer you steep, the more benefits. The amino acid L-theanine found in most teas improves memory and focus. Teas are chock-full of antioxidants that

- Help the body's ability to burn fat as fuel
- May aid cardiovascular health
- Protect against cancers
- Fight free radicals
- Improve bone mineral density and strength
- Reduce cortisol levels (when you drink up to 3 cups a day)
- Lower levels of inflammation

But, perhaps most important, we are finding that tea aids in gut health. Tea contains polyphenols (in the form of catechins in green tea and theaflavins and thearubigins in black tea),[4] which support the growth of good gut bacteria, such as bifidobacteria and lactobacilli, while combating bad bacteria including *C. difficile* (C. diff), *E. coli*, and salmonella, as well as improving symptoms of peptic ulcer disease (PUD) and inflammatory bowel disease (IBD).[5] Although green tea is often thought to have the most polyphenols, black tea has a similar amount, and in some cases even more. Greens, blacks, whites, and oolongs are all full of benefits, so don't stress over the dizzying array of teas out there — green over black, fruity over spicy, calming over energizing — they're all good.

Stressed out? Tea also contains theanine, a compound that has been shown to reduce the release of cortisol. If you drink tea, you will de-stress faster because your levels of cortisol will go down more quickly.[6] One last thing about tea: daily consumption of tea can reduce the risk of cognitive decline by 50 percent. While more research is needed to identify all of tea's benefits, the science already shows us just how good tea is for us. No wonder many cultures have been consuming tea for thousands of years. So drink up!

Try drinking 1–2 cups of tea in the morning. Especially if you are a coffee or diet soda drinker, drinking tea can be a healthful way to cut or eliminate those drinks that can be hard on digestion. Add warming spices to black tea with a touch of stevia (and maybe a splash of coconut milk) for a delicious chai (see my recipe for my Go-to Hormone-Balancing Chai Latte on page 224). If caffeine is an issue for you, you can try a decaffeinated variety.

Water, Agua, l'Eau

In whatever language, water, plain and simple, does the body good. Our bodies are composed of about 60 percent water, so I don't need to tell you how important it is to keep hydrated. But I will tell you a few H_2O facts that you may not know.

As water travels through your system, it flushes out toxins and keeps everything moving along, which in turn helps keep our gut bacteria balanced. Inadequate water intake is a common culprit in constipation and, believe or not, water retention (think feeling bloated and puffy). And our brains are greatly affected by our water intake: studies show that even mild dehydration (1–3 percent of body weight) can impair many aspects of brain functions, such as disruptions in mood and cognitive functioning.[7] Dehydration also increases cortisol.

Upping your water intake is a relatively easy change and certainly doesn't cost anything. Keep a glass or bottle (of non-BPA plastic, glass, or stainless steel!) of water by you at all times. I suggest drinking an 225-ml glass of water every morning, and keeping a glass by your bed at night. Drink it warm too. Warm water takes less energy to digest and stimulates digestion while detoxing the system and aiding food through the digestive tract. Drinking water, especially warm water on an empty stomach, is one of the best things you can do for digestion.

ENERGY BUSTER

Sorry, wine lovers, but this is for you. As you already know, I recommend limiting your alcohol intake. I know studies have shown that alcohol can be beneficial for reducing inflammation,[8] gut hormones, and energy levels. It's just got to be in the right amount — and quality matters. Red wine (and dark chocolate) includes those

---

wonderful polyphenols, but its benefits will be canceled out if you drink it (or, in the case of chocolate, eat it) to excess. Alcohol can increase estrogen levels and disrupt progesterone levels, causing a hormone imbalance, and there also could be increased chances of developing certain cancers, so there is a delicate balance of benefits and risks depending on how much you drink — and everybody is different. So drink to your health, but don't overdo it — no more than five drinks max a week. Wine is no better than hard alcohol — the important factor here is sugar. Stay away from sugary alcohol and premade mixes.

Other Superfoods

I pore over medical studies and health articles about superfoods, nutrients, and vitamins for the latest info to recommend to patients. I don't recommend anything unless it's backed by science and I feel absolutely confident that it's worth your time and money. Here are my favorites. Many of the superfoods listed here are spices that have anti-inflammatory properties, along with other medical benefits. They are also relatively inexpensive, making them easier to consume regularly (at least three times per week). You should eat these as part of a balanced whole-food, plant-based diet. They are easy to sprinkle on greens, add to smoothies, or to take in supplement form.

- *Cardamom:* This aromatic spice is known to have many anti-inflammatory properties and is packed with antioxidants; it's also known to aid digestion and help lessen the symptoms of a cold. If that's not enough, it also helps freshen your breath: studies show that cardamom may help fight bacteria in the mouth, a common cause of bad breath, cavities, and gum disease.[9]
- *Chia seeds:* The combination of omega-3 fatty acids, protein, and fiber makes chia seeds an anti-inflammatory powerhouse. One tablespoon of chia offers more calcium than a glass of milk. It's also full of antioxidants![10] Rich in fiber, they are also great for

weight loss. My favorite way to eat them is to soak them so they get a gel-like consistency. You can add soaked chia to practically anything: I like to add 2 tablespoons soaked for 15 minutes to smoothies or drink it with water, stevia, and lemon.

- *Cinnamon:* This yummy spice is one of the richest sources of antioxidants of any spice, and it is known to reduce inflammation. A good source of manganese, iron, and calcium, cinnamon lowers blood sugar and triglyceride levels and also reduces sugar and chocolate cravings. Add it to smoothies, oatmeal, tea, and even coffee for an extra dose of flavor.

- *Garlic:* Garlic has been shown to reduce inflammation, lower blood pressure, and treat colds. It can also reduce the risk of various cancers such as stomach, colon, lung, and breast. Garlic was recently repopularized by self-help author-podcaster Tim Ferriss, who says it helped him lose weight. Raw is best, but if you can't fathom eating it raw, extracts are available. To get the most benefit, let it sit out for about 20 minutes after chopping before using.

- *Ginger:* I'm not talking about sexy (former) Prince Harry. Ginger contains gingerol, a powerful anti-inflammatory and antioxidant. It has been shown to reduce muscle pain, improve cognitive function, and may have anti-diabetic properties by lowering fasting blood sugar. It certainly helps digestion by aiding the speed that the stomach empties after eating, and it can relieve gas, bloating, stomachache, indigestion, and nausea. To incorporate more ginger into your diet, drink it in a tea or grate it into . . . well, just about anything: stir-fry, vegetables, soups, burgers, roasts, eggs, muffins, oatmeal, smoothies, and desserts.

- *Ground flaxseeds:* Flaxseeds can help control your blood sugar and potentially inhibit certain cancers, such as prostate and breast. Just 2 tablespoons of ground flaxseed contain more than 140 percent of the daily value of the inflammation-reducing omega-3 fatty acids as well as more lignans, a cancer-fighting plant chemical, than any other plant food on the planet.[11] Additionally, they offer a good dose of soluble fiber. Try adding 2–3 tablespoons to your daily smoothie or over a salad.

- *Pepper:* Cayenne and other hot peppers (containing capsaicin) relieve aches and soreness, improve circulation, and aid heart health. Cayenne is also known as an appetite suppressant, so indulge, as long as you can take the heat! Black pepper has antibacterial properties and is rich in manganese, iron, potassium, chromium, vitamin C, vitamin K, and fiber. Interestingly, black pepper stimulates our taste buds, signaling hydrochloric acid secretion, which improves digestion.
- *Spirulina:* Spirulina is great for fighting inflammation, with tons of amino acids and antioxidants for immune support. It's also a great source of protein and a source of vegan B_{12} (a B vitamin sourced primarily in meat). The taste is a bit strong for some people, but the benefits, especially for plant-based eaters, are well worth it. I recommend getting the powder and adding a teaspoon into a smoothie or sprinkle on a salad.
- *Turmeric/curcumin:* Turmeric is a star in the spice world because of its anti-inflammatory properties. It has even been used in cancer trials because of its healing properties. Curcumin is the medicinal compound contained in turmeric. It has been shown to be effective in helping treat conditions like cancers, arthritis, and neurodegenerative diseases. It's also an effective pain reliever, rivaling over-the-counter pain relievers. Recent studies have also indicated that turmeric is a promising treatment for Alzheimer's too, as it can break down amyloid-beta plaques, a leading indicator of Alzheimer's.[12]

A Note on Spices

When I was researching spices, I realized that conventional spices can contain high levels of pesticides and other chemicals. This is especially true if they are produced in big factories. Opt for organic when you can.

As we know, a huge portion of the immune system lies in the gut. Using curry powder or raw turmeric can boost it. Turmeric is best eaten with black pepper and oil, because you absorb more of the active ingredient, curcumin, that way. Even just a little pinch of pepper — ½₀th of a teaspoon — can significantly boost bioavailability up to 2,000 percent. Try adding a half spoonful in hot water with a sprinkle of black pepper and a few drops of olive or coconut oil, or add it to your green (vegetable) juice — just make sure to add a few drops of oil and black pepper.

Don't Forget

Now you have my list of top superfoods, but here are some other star players to keep in mind:

Omega-3s

Omega-3s are good-for-you fats that are essential for optimum health. Why all the hubbub about omega-3s? Let me count the ways:

1. Support overall health and disease prevention
2. Support mental and behavioral health
3. Increase neuronal growth in the frontal cortex of the brain
4. Keep dopamine levels high
5. Decrease inflammation in the body and the brain
6. Reduce insulin resistance
7. Decrease risk of heart disease
8. Help with sleep issues

What are good sources of omega-3s? Fish and fish oil (mackerel, salmon, sardines, herring, anchovies), cod liver oil, flaxseed and flax oil, chia, hemp, shrimp, oysters, caviar, and some vegetables (cauliflower, brussels sprouts). The best way to boost omega-3s is to cut down on sources of omega-6s in your diet (grains, most animal products, and vegetable oils) and by eating more omega-3 foods to help tip that balance. If you take fish oil or a vegetarian-alternative omega-3 supplement, look for one with EPA and DHA, long-chain fatty acids that together help decrease inflammation.

Magnesium-Rich and Chromium-Rich Foods

Soil depletion, which robs foods of its important nutrients, an unbalanced gut microbiome that can't sufficiently absorb minerals, and poor diet can result in magnesium and chromium deficiencies. Adding foods rich in these two crucial minerals to your diet can aid energy levels, digestion, and combat cravings.

MAGNESIUM

- Optimizes energy expenditure, metabolism regulation, and work performance
- Aids insulin resistance
- Reduces sugar and carb cravings
- Regulates hormones
- Helps neurotransmitter release

FOODS HIGH IN MAGNESIUM

- Cacao
- Dark leafy greens (especially spinach and chard)
- Nuts and seeds (especially pumpkin seeds and almonds)
- Seafood
- Avocado
- Yogurt, kefir
- Black beans
- Figs

CHROMIUM

- Boosts the effectiveness of insulin
- Is crucial for keeping blood sugar stable
- Directly prevents carbohydrate cravings

FOODS HIGH IN CHROMIUM

- Broccoli
- Barley
- Oats
- Pork
- Green beans

- Tomatoes
- Dark leafy greens
- Black pepper

Soil Depletion

There is some research that over-farming, pesticides, and fertilizers have caused soil to be less nutritious, which in turn means plants grown in this soil are less nutritious. Studies that compared data from the US Department of Agriculture from the years 1950 and 1999 on 43 different vegetables and fruits found "reliable declines" in the amount of protein, calcium, phosphorus, iron, riboflavin (vitamin B_2), and vitamin C.[13] The jury is still out, but this is why eating organic is so important, if you can afford it. To get the most out of your fruits and veggies, go local and organic.

SUPPLEMENTS AREN'T ALL THAT

You'd think we could just have a plateful of supplements and be done with our nutrient intake for the day, right? Wrong. I don't recommend taking loads of supplements.

Here's why: Supplementing pales in comparison to eating nutritionally dense foods, because supplements don't include phytochemicals and phytonutrients that are vital for our health. There are literally thousands of phytochemicals in a stalk of broccoli that aren't in a supplement. You don't need phytochemicals to survive on a day-to-day basis like you do vitamins and minerals, but you do need them to keep your immune system operating optimally. When immunity is robbed of phytonutrients, you can't stave off inflammation as effectively. So taking supplements, even those that purportedly reduce inflammation, may be counterproductive for decreasing chronic inflammation if you use them instead of eating healthy greens.

However, in our modern world, we are deprived of adequate levels of certain nutrients that make supplementation necessary. Why? We simply aren't able to get necessary levels of everything through diet alone because our soil is less mineral-rich than it used to be (and hence our food is less nutritious), and we don't get adequate exposure to the sun that's needed for vitamin D production. Also modern farming and agricultural practices have changed our diet and decreased our nutrient intake. For this reason, I do supplement high-quality B and D vitamins, omega-3s and adaptogens, but I look to food sources for all other nutrition needs. Spend a little extra on organic produce, protein, and grains that contain more vitamins, minerals, and phytochemicals and eat a variety of foods, and you won't need a ton of supplements, either.

❧

I talked earlier in the book about why supplements aren't always what they are marketed to be, so just remember that if and when you do use supplements, know that you get what you pay for and opt for viable manufacturers like Thorne or Source Naturals. Do your research on sites like consumerlabs.com, and talk to your health care practitioner (so long as you are certain he or she isn't pushing a product for a kickback).

WHAT TO AVOID OR LIMIT

Now you know all of the good stuff to eat — here's a look at the stuff you want to avoid or limit on this plan.

Processed Foods

You know what these are: they come in a package, and they have *a lot* of ingredients (usually with ten different ways of listing sugar). Avoid/eliminate anything with the following:

- *Artificial preservatives:* If your food does not spoil in a week, it's because of preservatives! These additives extend the shelf life of foods, but think about it: when something keeps your food "fresh" for that long, there has to be something not natural about it. Some keywords to look for include sodium nitrate, sodium benzoate, BHA, BHT, and TBHQ. The International Agency for Research on Cancer (IARC) has classified nitrates as probably carcinogenic.[14] I suggest eating clean, whole foods — you'll avoid preservatives altogether with its label-free packaging.
- *Excess sodium:* Canned foods, frozen foods, and dry powders are the worst offenders.
- *Added sugar (and hidden sugar):* High-fructose corn syrup, dextrose, cane syrup solids. (Note: Manufacturers can be sneaky and will list sugar under different names so that there can be 4–8 types of sugar. This means that your "healthy" granola bar may be up to 80 percent sugar, but the first — and most prominent — ingredient can still be listed as "oats.")
- *Hydrogenated oils:* Found in margarine, vegetable shortening, and packaged goods, they contain harmful trans fats.
- *MSG, or monosodium glutamate:* A food additive in many prepared foods, it is known to cause headaches and to worsen asthma.
- *Sulfites:* Commonly used as preservatives in processed foods, they can cause a variety of problems, from dermatitis to diarrhea to asthma.[15]
- *FD&C artificial colors:* Added to all types of foods to enhance appearance. Whether these dyes are safe is highly controversial — many believe them to be toxic. While the FDA approves their use, many European countries limit them.

A good rule of thumb is to shop at a place like Whole Foods, which bans most of these ingredients, health food stores, or a farmers market, where foods don't need to have a long shelf life.

Omega-6 Oils

Here's the CliffsNotes version on omega-6 and omega-3 fats and oils: There is a natural balance of omega-6s and omega-3s in a healthy, whole-food diet. But in our current diet, which relies heavily on processed foods, most Americans are ingesting way too many omega-6 fats from the overuse of cheap, processed oils in the feed we give to livestock (instead of the omega-3 grass they used to eat). (Conversely, we have a decreased consumption of omega-3-rich foods like fish and vegetables.) When we eat these omega-6-filled foods, the omega-6 reacts with insulin to create inflammation, which is a disaster because, as you know, a high-carb diet (aka the SAD, or standard American diet) pumps too much insulin into the bloodstream, creating a volatile cesspool of inflammation and adipose tissue (fat).

Omega-6 oils include

- Corn oil
- Safflower oil
- Cottonseed oil
- Soy oil
- Vegetable oil (I know, it sounds good for you)
- Canola oil
- Sunflower oil
- Palm oil
- Most grapeseed oils (sorry, this one too)

Another good rule of thumb is to stick to the following oils: olive oil (unheated or at low heat), avocado oil or coconut oil for high-heat cooking, and walnut/pistachio/pumpkin seed/flax oil for smoothies, yogurt, and oatmeal.

Food Sensitivities

Food sensitivities, as opposed to a food allergy, are hard to pinpoint, although they do wreak havoc on the gut, create inflammation, and disrupt hormone balance. Gluten and dairy are in close competition for the award for most common food sensitivity.

Wheat/Gluten

Studies support that in about 90 percent of the population, wheat can initiate leaky gut. In up to 80 percent of the population, gluten causes inflammation. What exactly is gluten? Gluten is a protein found in wheat; in fact, it's the primary protein in wheat, making up 80 percent of its protein content.

Good rule of thumb: Avoid gluten and wheat, and if you are trying to lose weight or fix autoimmune issues, then avoid all grains for the next 30 days. Because of the decreased nutritional value and loss of diversity in grains, they should be a small part of our diet.

Most Dairy

Conventional dairy products, like processed foods or non-organic cheese and milk, can contain high levels of omega-6s because the dairy cows are fed an all-grain diet. Worse, conventionally raised dairy cows are fed hormones to increase milk production and are given antibiotics to keep them "healthy" in their crowded farming environments. It's no surprise that these hormones and antibiotics can disrupt our hormone balance when we eat conventional dairy, creating sickness and weight gain. To boot, pasteurization — the process of treating dairy products with high heat to destroy pathogens — destroys the enzymes in raw dairy that would help us digest it more easily.

So if you tolerate dairy, there is no reason to avoid or eliminate it during this program. If you're unsure, avoid all dairy for a month and then slowly reintroduce the healthier forms of dairy like fermented, full-fat, or raw dairy and see how you feel (see page 93).

THE NUTTY WORLD OF PLANT-BASED MILK (AND CHEESE) ALTERNATIVES

The explosion of nut milks on the scene is enough to confuse anyone. The dairy-free option is surely a welcome substitute for those who are lactose intolerant or wanting to steer clear of cow milk for its possible hormones. More and more types seem to be popping up — soy milk was first, soon eclipsed by almond milk, then cashew, coconut, and oat milk. All have their fans, but when looking at the most beneficial in terms of nutrition, it seems almond and cashew milk are best for calcium and vitamins D and E. They are lower in protein than regular milk, and with almond milk you also have to be concerned about the environmental impact, for one glass of almond milk uses 74 litres of water to produce. In terms of dietary health, whatever you choose, read your labels. Many nut milks add sugar, salt, and gums for flavoring, so choose unsweetened. If soy is your choice, pay particular attention to what is discussed below. Soy has isoflavones — plant compounds that mimic estrogen; isoflavones can wreak havoc with your hormones and lead to all sorts of issues, and they have been linked to breast cancer.

Bottom line: don't get caught up in the details. If it tastes good and your body doesn't react to it, stick to your favorites — whether it is dairy or nondairy. My number one rule: buy as local, organic, and homemade as possible.

To Meat or Not to Meat

Meat has been traditionally thought of as part of a healthy, well-balanced diet since it has the most protein (and iron) for the buck. Meat on the daily dinner table has been as American as apple pie for decades. But the rise of vegetarianism and veganism is catching on, and for good reason. I could write ad nauseam about the humane and environmental impacts of commercial meat production, but that is another book. Here, I want you to consider the health implications of eating meat.

First and foremost, processed meat (think hot dogs, deli turkey, roast beef, pepperoni, chicken nuggets, sausage, and ham) is full of antibiotics, pesticides, and preservatives that have been linked with inflammation, cancer, heart disease, high blood pressure, and a whole host of other diseases. While the jury is out, some research shows that antibiotics and hormones pumped into commercial meat to prevent infections and promote growth are also thought to be negative to our health and may cause antibiotic resistance.[16]

Some meats are high in saturated fat, which can raise LDL cholesterol levels. Leaner meats, like chicken, have fewer saturated fats than red meat.

Meat contains insulin-like growth factor 1. IGF-1 is a hormone naturally found in animals, including humans, that promotes growth. When IGF-1 is consumed, not only is this hormone itself taken in, but it stimulates the body's own production of the hormone.[17] All this excess IGF-1 can promote cancer growth.

When meat is cooked at high temperatures, the compounds known as polycyclic aromatic hydrocarbons, heterocyclic amines, and advanced glycans are formed and can be carcinogenic.[18] These compounds are also pro-inflammatory, pro-oxidative, and contributive to chronic disease. Meat also contains a compound called N-glycolylneuraminic acid (Neu5Gc) that has been shown to promote chronic inflammation.[19]

Red meat can also raise the levels of TMAO (trimethylamine N-oxide) — a by-product formed by the gut during digestion, which has been found to increase the risk of cardiovascular disease, including heart attacks and strokes.[20] (Take note, as this is far from conclusive, and there has been some research showing that TMAO is helpful in some ways.[21])

What does this all mean? If you eat meat, avoid processed meat, do your research, and read your labels; find out as much as possible about the meat you are consuming. Go organic, grass-fed, hormone-free, antibiotic-free as much as possible. All the meals in this plan are animal free, but if you want to add meat, I suggest adhering to a plant-based diet for 90 percent of it; if you want an organic, grass-fed burger or eggs once or twice a week, go for it (limiting it to stay within the 10 percent parameter of the WTF plan).

What About Eggs?

If you can tolerate them, eggs are good in moderation. Rich in protein and omega-3s, eggs used to get a bad rap for being high in cholesterol, but recently the *British Medical Journal* concluded that moderate egg consumption is not associated with increased risk of coronary heart disease. So if you don't have a history of cardiac disease, feel free to crack one open —just make sure they are within that 10 percent window. And buy cage-free and certified organic.[22]

How About Fish?

Fish, on the other hand, is an excellent and healthier source of protein. Studies indicate that certain fish can be quite anti-inflammatory. In fact, a few studies have found fish oil to be as good as high-dose NSAIDs like ibuprofen for pain and inflammation. Fish is also a rich source of omega-3 fatty acids, which have been shown over and over again to not only stop inflammation but to heal it. If you like fish, make sure it's an omega-3 type — mackerel, lake trout, herring, sardines, albacore tuna, and salmon are all good choices. Do watch out for how the fish was raised: wild-caught is better than farmed because their diet is more diverse. Fish can have an excessive amount of mercury, pesticide residues, and other toxins depending on their source.[23] Again, read your labels and go organic and as fresh as possible.

Soy

As a health professional, I get asked about soy a lot, since it's one of the most common food allergens in the Westernized world. But it is also a great source of protein (100 grams of soy contain 17 grams of protein!) and is what's known as a "complete protein," which means it has all of the amino acids that our body needs to convert a food to protein in one source. Because of this rare trait in a plant-based food, soy is considered equivalent in protein quality to animal proteins, and hence a staple of vegetarian and vegan diets.

But the soy landscape has gotten more confusing recently. A few years ago, soy manufacturers funded a PR push after some studies showed that it helped ease some menopausal symptoms such as hot flashes. But then the pendulum swung the other way, and soy became the scapegoat for almost everything under the sun, including cancer.[24]

If you're adopting a plant-based lifestyle, this is an even trickier topic, since you're faced with soy in practically every product in the vegetarian section of your grocery store. It's difficult to completely remove soy from your diet as it's in so many things; you'd have to drastically move away from all mainstream food choices to avoid it.

But what is the real risk of moderate consumption? And why is there so much polarized information? I've boiled it all down to the top six facts you need to know about soy:

1. Some people think because soy contains isoflavones, which are similar to estrogen, it may be bad for us. Isoflavones can block the more potent natural estrogens from binding to the estrogen receptor, but they can also provide a host of benefits: they can lower cholesterol and the risk of cardiovascular disease and some cancers. So, the topic is much more complex than is usually presented in the media.

2. High consumption of processed soy *may* contribute to breast cancer. This, to me, is the thorniest issue. Some articles support the idea that soy contributes to breast cancer, but most of them studied soy consumption at extremely high levels, and most of them had the participants eat processed soy. Also, many of them were animal studies. Quite a few sources such as the Cleveland Clinic and the Mayo Clinic say that soy in moderation and in unprocessed forms does not correlate with increased risk of breast cancer.[25]

3. Soy allegedly affects your thyroid, especially if you already have hypothyroidism. If so, avoid consuming more than two daily servings of soy.
4. More than 90 percent of soy produced in the United States is genetically modified, and there is continued use of pesticides during farming, most notably a weed-killer known as Roundup. A concentrate of the chemical glyphosate, this product is known to be an endocrine disruptor and has been attributed to a number of health issues such as cancer, liver damage, and heart disease. Also, in the US, there are no regulations that separate GMO soy fields from non-GMO fields, so the non-GMO soy plants can get contaminated.
5. A lot of soy is often highly processed. Like wheat, part of the problem with soy is that it often comes in the processed form of snacks, cakes, and meat alternatives. In my practice, I find that cutting out soy and wheat from the diet is beneficial, not just because you're cutting out inflammatory foods, but because it forces you to cut out processed foods such as cakes, cookies, energy bars, and other junk food.
6. Soybean oil is processed with hexane — a by-product of gasoline refining — in its initial stages of extraction. If you choose organic soy products or unprocessed soy (like edamame), you don't have to worry about hexane use.

Okay, so what's the final verdict? Soy is fine — actually more than fine for those who are looking at it as a source of protein — as long as you avoid the processed forms of it. I enjoy whole organic soy a few times a week, so feel free to do the same. Check ingredient labels and steer clear of soy powder and stick to organic, non-GMO, sprouted and/or fermented soy. Think sprouted organic tofu, edamame, and fermented soy like miso.

Bad Fats

Something happened right around the end of the 1970s: fat became a villain. Actually it became *the* villain — the root of heart disease, obesity, and early death according to just about every publication and medical journal. Hence the low-fat craze began, and we turned away from butter, full-fat dairy, oils, and animal fat. The problem is that we replaced fat with carbohydrates and sugar. And the processed foods that were labeled "low fat" were just as bad as fattening foods (if not worse). Our blood sugar and insulin levels shot up. Contrary to the theory that low-fat, high-carbohydrate diets would make us lean and healthy, we got fatter and sicker, leaving us with our current epidemic of obesity and metabolic disorders.

Don't be afraid of fat — just eat healthy fats and avoid the harmful ones. The fats that you should steer clear of are animal fats, vegetable oils, peanut oil, canola oil, soybean oil, cottonseed oil, sunflower oil, margarine, shortening, or "spreads" — all of which are high in omega-6 fats. Your friendly fats include whole coconut, avocados, olive oil, and other healthy sources of saturated fat that can diminish inflammation. When you eat whole fats like nuts, avocado, and coconut, your body feels satisfied and there is not such an insulin spike as when you eat sugar. That leads to less fat storage and less inflammation. Adding oily fish and fish oil, which contain polyunsaturated omega-3 fats, to your diet is one of the easiest ways to help balance your hormones and lower inflammation. If you're vegan, omega-3 fats are also found in algae oil and (in lesser amounts) in chia seeds, flax, and walnuts.

Artificial Sweeteners/Diet Soda

Some evidence suggests that diet soda disrupts insulin signaling and therefore can lead to weight gain, especially around the belly. Abdominal fat is associated with increased cardiovascular disease, inflammation, and insulin resistance. Sugar-free products, especially sodas, are sweetened at 200–600 times the sweetness of sugar. Artificial sweeteners confuse the body into thinking it has consumed something super sweet, which in turn leads to cravings for sweeter and sweeter things.

Interestingly, artificial sweeteners actually *overstimulate* the brain's reward centers, which are activated when we do something pleasurable or eat something sweet and "addictive." This changes the way we process sweet "rewards," so we need more and more sweetness and stronger flavors to satisfy our cravings. Artificial sweeteners can make us crave artificially flavored sweet foods like cookies, cupcakes, and so on, which makes healthier, less-processed staples like sweet potatoes and broccoli seem bland to our now-overstimulated taste buds.

Evidence suggests (but is nonconclusive) that artificial sweeteners can lead to insulin resistance, leptin imbalance, and glucose intolerance because they change our gut microbiome, leading to weight gain and disease.

❧

Another good rule of thumb: ideally *eliminate* all artificial sweeteners and diet soda. If you must have a sweetener, organic raw stevia, erythritol, or monk fruit is okay. Have a diet soda habit? Try sparkling water or lemonade with a hint of stevia and cayenne pepper.

Protein — Too Much of a Good Thing?

Protein is overrated. To me, having a really high-protein diet is just as bad as a high-sugar diet. I can hear the collective "But why? I thought protein is so good for us?" It sure is: protein, made out of essential amino acids, is key for bone and muscle development, cell repair, and brainpower. So high-protein diets are becoming increasingly popular because, in theory, getting a lot of protein sounds good, right? Why not get the most protein you can if it is so important to our bodies? Well, there is something to be said about getting too much of a good thing. While the consensus is still out, research points to too much protein being not great for the body. For instance, the University of Eastern Finland tracked 2,400 middle-aged men for over 22 years and found that a high-protein diet resulted in a 49 percent greater risk of heart failure.[26] Other studies have shown that people who consume large amounts of protein, especially red and processed meat, are more likely to be obese and have increased risk of developing type 2 diabetes, heart issues, and colon cancer.[27]

Harvard researcher Dr. David Sinclair has shown that those who eat a lot of protein have lower NAD levels (small molecules essential to our metabolism), which, without getting too clinical, shuts off the mTOR pathway that promotes longevity.[28]

So let's break it down for the real world: On average, a man should get about 56 grams of protein per day while women should get 46 grams per day (0.8 grams of protein a day for each kilogram you weigh). Current USDA dietary guidelines suggest that adult men and women consume between 10 and 35 percent of their total calories from protein. (Each gram of protein contains four calories.)[29]

People on diets that are too high in protein show signs of the following:

- Increased risk of cardiovascular disease because of high levels of sulfur amino acids in protein
- Nutritional deficiencies or insufficient fiber, which can cause problems such as bad breath, headache, and constipation
- Impaired kidney function in people with kidney disease because the body may have trouble eliminating all the waste products of protein metabolism
- Altered pH balance, making the gut more acidic, which is thought to encourage cancerous growths

In the US, we tend to go "big" — supersized sodas, movie theater mega-complexes, and McMansions. And we tend to do that with our protein intake, too. While protein is absolutely essential for growth and cell repair, there is a downside in overdoing protein consumption. In the body, there is an opposition between growth and longevity, like a seesaw, and so we need to keep that seesaw in balance. The hormone insulin-like growth factor 1 (IGF-1), something that has a crucial role in childhood growth, can also play a role in how we age: it is thought that excess protein can cause too much production of IGF-1, which as we get older can cause growth of cancerous cells along with healthy ones.[30]

So when it comes to protein, quality should outweigh quantity. If you want protein, I say stick to plant-based foods like beans, chickpeas, tofu, nuts, and fish, if you eat it. If you are a meat eater, stay away from processed meats and limit your intake. A serving of grass-fed meat like chicken or fresh fish a couple times a week is okay. You can get adequate protein much easier than you think—you don't need those processed bars, protein powders, and muscle milk.

ENERGY BOOSTERS

Here is a good cheat sheet for all the foods that are high in anti-inflammatory properties.

- Garlic
- Beets
- Raw nuts
- Berries
- Tea
- Ginger
- Turmeric
- Flax seeds
- Cardamom
- Chia seeds
- Avocado
- Broccoli
- Pineapple
- Dandelion greens
- Coconut
- Spinach

THE NEW FOOD PYRAMID

Remember in elementary school when you learned about the food pyramid? Created by the Department of Health in the late twentieth century, the illustration showed recommended food allowances with proportions of what should be consumed in a day and how much.

Grains and carbs were on the bottom tier, indicating they should be the lion's share of daily food intake. The pyramid has been modified in recent years to change with the times, but not by much. Grains have switched places with fruits and veggies to become the second largest portion. If I were to redo the pyramid, prebiotic fiber in the form of vegetables would be at the bottom, along with water and anti-inflammatory spices like ginger and garlic. Then the next tier would be whole-food protein like tofu, nuts, and beans and whole-food fat like avocado and coconut. Next up would be whole-food carbohydrates (fruit, sweet potato, whole corn). On the tippy top would be processed junk like candy, cookies, and white bread (the 10 percent I allow in my plan).

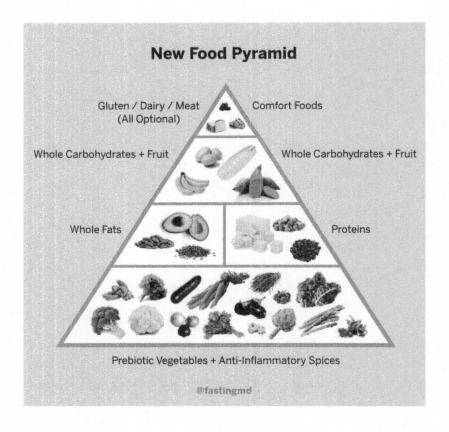

New Food Pyramid

Gluten / Dairy / Meat (All Optional) — Comfort Foods

Whole Carbohydrates + Fruit — Whole Carbohydrates + Fruit

Whole Fats — Proteins

Prebiotic Vegetables + Anti-Inflammatory Spices

@fastingmd

AND, OH YEAH, KEEP
STRESS LEVELS DOWN

Were you aware that your blood sugar rises when you become
stressed or anxious? If the answer is no, you're definitely not alone.

We have talked about stress a lot and how it causes major havoc
on our hormones, immune system, and the gut, so you know that
stress can be terrible for our overall health. But stress also has a direct impact on our blood sugar. Roughly 50 percent of Americans
are now either prediabetic or have full-blown type 2 diabetes, so it
is impossible to ignore that Americans have a blood sugar problem.
There has been an enormous amount of attention to the dangers of
sugars, simple carbs, and other foods that can contribute to insulin
resistance, but little has been said about the effect of stress on blood
sugar and how it might be worse than soda, candy, or white bread for
our bodies.

It's important to understand the connection between your stress
levels and your blood glucose for a few reasons. For starters, high
blood sugar can lead to many diseases, including obesity, diabetes,
and heart disease. In addition, even if you're trying to combat blood
sugar issues by adopting a low-carb diet, a keto diet, or an intermittent fasting plan, stress may be sabotaging your efforts by spiking
your blood sugar even when you're avoiding carbs or eating only fat
and protein.

How does this work exactly? Well, we have talked about how
when you're stressed your body activates its fight-or-flight physiological response. Part of this response involves your body releasing
blood sugar into your bloodstream so that you can use it immediately in an emergency situation. When you're always stressed, you

get a constant blood sugar release, which causes more insulin to be released as well.

This high insulin state, hyperinsulinemia, causes your body to try to force glucose back into cells. Insulin is also one of the hormones that signals your body to store fat, which explains why people often gain weight during a stressful time in their lives — even if they don't change their eating habits.

While all this occurs, the brain perceives the stress or anxiety and releases cortisol from the adrenals, and also releases blood sugar and causes the liver to regenerate glucose in a process called gluconeogenesis. Once the stressful event is over, the signal stops. This is fine if it occurs infrequently, but for most of us, this is happening a few times a week, daily, or even hourly. It can leave your body really confused and with a lot of unnecessary glucose floating around in the bloodstream that the muscles and body do not actually need.

This explains why people often have problems related to high blood sugar even when they're taking steps to clean up their diet and lifestyle. In fact, many experts — including me! — believe that stress and sleep have the largest impact on blood sugar levels. Maybe even more than the food you eat.

So what can you do about it? We can't avoid stress altogether, but I recommend taking note of the stress- and anxiety-provoking situations you encounter regularly. For me, working out VERY early in the morning (like 6 a.m.) has become too stressful and forces me to skimp on sleep. As someone who is trying to do everything I can to prevent diabetes, I decided the increased stress to get to the gym is not worth the benefit of that workout. Evaluate your life and make moves to reduce negative stress as much as possible. Your blood sugar will thank you for it.

AND GET YOUR SLEEP

Sleep is king, no one will deny that. It's key to improving any type of previous hormonal blockage or imbalance, and it is the last part of this plan to optimize the energy trifecta. Try to sleep 9–10 hours a night rather than just 6–8, and assess how you are feeling after a period of more rest. Use the two days on your extended gut rest to get into your PJs and catch up on your sleep — the extra zzz's make the fasting go faster, too. You may ask: *But do I really need that many hours of sleep?* Whether or not you feel it now, prolonged lack of sleep has the following effects:

- Decreases brainpower
- Weakens your immune response
- Kills your sex drive
- Increases cravings for carbohydrates and sugar
- Ages your skin
- Depletes your energy
- Puts you at risk for heart disease, diabetes, and some cancers
- Screws with your hormones

Maybe you're thinking, *But I get five hours of sleep a night, and I'm fine!* Sure, for now. But you might literally be taking years off your life, by denying your body and mind the sleep it needs.

A study from researchers in the UK found that people who went from 7 hours to 5 hours or less of sleep a night suffered a 1.7-fold increased risk of premature death from all causes. That suggests you are 1.7 times more likely to live a shortened life by not getting your 7+ hours a night. P.S. If you're thinking to yourself, *Really? I'm less likely to get hit by a bus?* Yes, you are.

Want to improve your productivity and boost your career? Sleep. Your ability to think, reason, react, and respond will slow with sleep deprivation. Cognitive functions, memory, perception, and creativity are compromised. Your emotions will be less regulated — that is, you will be cranky and tend to overreact. (*What do you mean, overreact?!*)

Researchers have actually likened sleep deprivation to being intoxicated on alcohol. And sleep affects the prefrontal cortex — that's the part of the brain that processes inhibition. So you'll be more likely to pick up things like junk food, cigarettes, or surf the internet instead of doing something productive or fulfilling. It also weakens your immune system, because certain immune cells peak when you sleep at night. Meaning, the less sleep you get, the more you are susceptible to illnesses like the common cold or more-serious diseases like diabetes, heart conditions, or cancer. Also brain disorders like dementia and Alzheimer's have been linked to lack of sleep and sleep apnea.

Lastly, your hormones depend on sleep. Take melatonin (the "sleep hormone"), for example. You've probably heard to pop a melatonin supplement if you can't sleep. Burning the midnight oil — staying awake, or being exposed to light when it's dark and you should be powering down — can throw off melatonin cycles and make it so melatonin is not being released normally. We know this affects sleep, but we are finding out that it may affect many more processes in the body than previously realized.

Key Takeaways About Melatonin

- It is only released in the dark/at night.
- It creates drowsiness.
- It aids in recovery from exercise.
- It has strong antioxidant effects — it actually may help strengthen the immune system.
- It helps with blood pressure regulation.
- It plays a role in the female reproductive cycle.

Another hormone affected by sleep? Insulin. This is the hormone that allows the body to use sugar from carbohydrates for energy or to store for future use. If there is too much sugar in the body, insulin stores it in liver and fat cells to restore balance. Not enough sugar, and insulin releases these stores. Too little sleep may cause insulin resistance, which means the body can't use insulin properly; blood sugar spikes, and so does the risk of chronic disease and obesity.

Okay, what about those hormones you don't hear as much about — like human growth hormone, leptin, and ghrelin? Yep, they are affected by sleep as well. The nightly production of leptin, which suppresses appetite, goes down with less sleep. The levels of ghrelin, which stimulates hunger and is secreted at night, increase an average of 15 percent in participants getting five hours of sleep versus eight hours. (Know how you tend to get hungry when you're tired? Well, now you know why.) Also released by the brain during sleep is human growth hormone, which promotes growth, cell reproduction and regeneration (i.e., anti-aging), cognitive function, and overall well-being. So if you are getting less sleep, you are getting less of this wonder hormone.

All right, are you convinced yet? Here are seven tips to start getting better zzz's in your life:

1. Change your mindset from "the strong only need 4 hours of sleep a night" to "I need at least 7 hours of sleep tonight or I am at risk of overeating, being groggy, cranky, and generally destroying my health and quality of life."
2. Make sure to always sleep in the dark, and get lots of light in the daytime. Hang blackout shades in your bedroom, and expose yourself to natural sunlight in the morning — for instance, exercise, work, or walk outside for a bit, if you can. Circadian rhythm, aka your internal clock or sleep-wake cycle, is controlled by an area of the brain that responds to light.
3. To the best of your ability, make your bed and bedroom for sleeping only. All other activities should be done somewhere else so that you unconsciously associate your bed with sleeping. If you watch TV, work, shop online, or eat in bed and have trouble sleeping, keep those activities out of your bed and bedroom.
4. Also, be sure to keep your bedroom cool at night. Cooler temperatures are close to our own internal body temperature (which drops to its lowest level when we sleep). Temperatures above or below this range seem to breed restless sleep. Temperatures of 60 to 68 degrees work best. Cold showers before bed help as well.
5. If your sleep is restless or you wake up at 3 a.m. and can't fall back to sleep, it's likely because your mind is racing — that is,

you are experiencing anxiety or mental stress. Listening to meditation or relaxation guides or sounds can be helpful. Do what you can to not bring your stresses to bed with you.

6. Herbal tea can also be useful. I'm not necessarily talking chamomile, though that works for some. If you really can't sleep and don't have adverse side effects, try relaxing/sedating herbs like Sleepytime tea, valerian root, kava kava, and magnesium. However, be aware that if you consistently use these supplements to sleep, you will have trouble in the long term sleeping without them, so don't rely on these alone — make additional changes to your bedroom and bedtime routine to support healthier sleep habits.

7. Avoid eating three hours before bed. This optimizes blood sugar and insulin, contributing to not only more restful sleep but overall better health. Eating too close to bedtime, late at night, or in the middle of the night desynchronizes your internal clock, which leads to sleeplessness and weight gain.

Well, that was a lot of information to digest (pun not intended). But here are the bare essentials to remember. Working within the timeline of circadian fasting, the WTF plan centers around three essential parts: 6–8 servings of vegetables daily, prebiotic foods, and hormone-balancing tea. And I walk you through how to put this all together in the next chapter.

❧

I'll leave you with this. You are what you eat. So let's move forward onto how exactly to clean up your diet with more veggies and fewer processed foods and sugar.

8

Get with the WTF Plan

I WAS THE PERFECT EXAMPLE of a fasting failure. When I first tried IF about five years ago, I jumped right into it because I am eternally that A+ overachiever. I ate so little the first day that I couldn't sleep at night from crazy hunger pangs. By the second day, I was already feeling fatigued and didn't sleep well. I was having trouble exercising properly, and I was pushing through my day to the point where I was not functioning. By the third morning, I was so tired and cranky I barked at my husband, couldn't think clearly at work, and grossly overate during my window of eating. I felt depleted — and yes, still starving! I quit after a week.

But a few months later, as more research was published about the benefits of fasting, I was reminded that this may be the key to both energy and long-term health, and I tried again. This time I made small and gradual changes, I saw how the *right kind* of fasting (tailored for a woman: see sidebar on page 192) changed my body and the way I eat and, more important, how I feel. Since then, I have recommended my fasting plan hundreds of times over to family, friends, and patients, and now I offer it to you.

Are you ready to feel revitalized, rejuvenated, *and* get out of calorie-counting hell? The following plan will give you the necessary tools to take control of your energy levels and change your health for the better. This two-week jump-start plan is something you can rinse and repeat and extend, or you can modify it to your lifestyle — don't worry, I will give you tips and advice on how to do that.

The WTF plan combines my circadian fasting with healthy hormone-balancing and energy-pumping foods. This combination will align you with your internal clock and make your body work like a well-oiled machine — as nature intended. It will improve gut health, which will in turn balance out hormones and, more important, make your energy skyrocket. You will finally be able to take control of your personal health and wellness journey. The best part? I made all the mistakes and took all the wrong turns already, so you don't have to experience all the challenges and pitfalls that I encountered!

My circadian fasting takes advantage of our own body's internal clock and the power of the sun and our own circadian rhythms. This plan is different from what you read about in other IF plans on the internet, combining age-old wisdom with cutting-edge science. It involves restricting your food intake to 9 or 12 hours a day, and tailoring that window of time so that you have an early dinner instead of skipping breakfast. Studies show that it is better to have an early dinner than it is to skip your breakfast, which may cause inflammation.[1]

Syncing eating with your circadian rhythms can level out insulin levels and increase human growth hormone levels, which lead to weight loss, increased cellular repair, and can even help heal epigenetic changes that can prevent future diseases and illness. Also, your diabetic risk decreases because your blood sugar levels have stabilized and reduced.

It's great for your digestion — it gives your body a break so your gut can repair and reset. Bonus points: you will sleep better, wake up rested, and your skin will glow. Under this approach, eating is timed within a 9- to 12-hour daytime window in conjunction with meals that are yummy, filling, and easy to make. Combine circadian fasting with timed sleep-wake cycles as well as exposure to sunlight each day for a balanced, healthy, new *you*.

While this program is not primarily used for weight loss, gut rest (if done correctly and regularly) will indeed change your body composition through loss of fat mass and weight as well as improve markers of disease that are associated with carrying excess weight, such as blood pressure and cholesterol levels. Another key reason intermittent fasting works (in addition to the metabolic switching) is because it helps you reduce caloric intake. Your eating period is reduced to a smaller window, and you will be taking in less food and fewer calories as long as you stay on a healthy diet and do not overeat during your eating window. It may take 1–3 months to start seeing weight loss, but you will definitely feel mentally and physically better even if you don't see an immediate change on the scale.

There is vast evidence that links weight loss with intermittent fasting:

- Regular food restriction can lead to weight-loss plateaus as the body adjusts to lower caloric consumption; intermittent fasting prevents the body from adjusting and burning less fat, because you toggle between low-calorie and normal eating.
- A 2015 meta-analysis of 40 studies about intermittent fasting shows that participants shed 10 pounds over a 10-week period. A second study demonstrated that adults participating in alternate-day fasting lost 13 pounds over an 8-week period.
- Intermittent fasting also targets and reduces visceral fat (internal fat packed deep around your abdominal organs). A different and more targeted study demonstrated that people were able to shed between 4 and 7 percent of visceral fat through intermittent fasting over a 6-month period.

I guarantee you will see change quickly when you follow the WTF plan: although there are 100 trillion bacteria in our gut, studies show that this crowded microbiome can change in as little as three days. However, real, long-lasting change takes more time, so while this is laid out in a two-week plan, this is not a quick fix—this is a lifetime plan. The longer you do it, the better you will feel. This is not about losing 10–20 pounds. This is about boosting your energy to live a better life. You want more energy for the rest of your life, right? This is your forever diet: a program that can keep you energized for 6 months, 3 years, 20 years, and more.

A SNAPSHOT OF THE WTF PLAN

Although we will provide you with meal ideas along the way, there are guidelines you should follow for every one of the next 14 days. From what we know about the microbiome, eating fresh, fermented, real food is the key to a healthy gut. So that means a diet that's predominantly plant-based, as well as gluten-free and dairy-free. But I want this plan to be flexible. If you can tolerate gluten, meat, and dairy, you can certainly adjust the plan. Just make high-quality choices: read your labels and buy as fresh and as organic as possible. My rule of thumb: follow 90 percent of my plan, eating mostly a plant-based diet, with prebiotic foods at every meal, leaving about 10 percent wiggle room for your own tastes.

This can be really easy to do if you batch cook once a week. (Sundays are a great option for most people.) I recommend roasting prebiotic-rich vegetables like asparagus, dandelion greens, onions, garlic, and Jerusalem artichokes. Eat them throughout the week to ensure you're getting high amounts of prebiotics; this will strengthen the gut-immune-hormone connection. Aim for about 5–7 servings of vegetables a day. Remember, the more diverse the plants you consume, the more diverse your microbiota will be. While the goal is to keep your diet very plant heavy, you can incorporate modest amounts of animal foods like eggs or fish if you wish.

It is also vital for you to get adequate sleep and manage your stress as you begin the program. Work on your mindset and your sleep, sync your daily routine according to circadian rhythms, and manage your physical and emotional stress. This plan is a hormetic stressor (as is all intermittent fasting). Any positive steps you take toward your gut health will be negated if you are stressed and tired. Along with a clear timetable of when you can eat, there are also certain foods and drinks you should be focusing on — and avoiding. During your fasting periods, you can have the following:

- Water
- Black coffee
- Tea
- A touch of stevia (or monk fruit or erythritol) is okay, just use sparingly. Avoid artificial sweeteners and diet drinks as they can break your fast and trigger a higher production of insulin.[2]

What Is a Hormetic Stressor?

This entire program of IF is in itself a hormetic stressor, meaning it puts your body in a state of hormesis — a physiological stress on your body that in turn helps its overall response system. There is convincing research that mice on calorie-restrictive diets showed promising longevity and health gains.[3] The best analogy to explain hormesis is weight training: When you work out, you are putting stress on your muscles to the point of fatigue, and then you let them rest. During that rest, the muscles go into repair mode, making them, and your body, stronger.

With IF, the restricted caloric intake is a stress to your body, and your body's response system, like that of all organisms, wants to maintain homeostasis; doing so makes your body stronger and more resistant in an effort to keep that equilibrium.[4] As a result, hormesis turns on all the longevity and metabolic pathways, lowering your cholesterol, blood sugar levels, and insulin sensitivity, among other indicators — all the signs of good health.

Simply put, a small amount of well-timed stress is good for you.

BREAKING THE FAST

First and foremost, you don't want to break a fast with an all-you-can-eat breakfast — fiber first. When your fast is over and it's time for your first meal of the day, it's important to take a restrained approach to eating — even though you're hungry. You'll want to refuel with easy-to-digest foods and beverages that are nutrient-dense. Additionally, plan ahead and practice "mindful eating" — a no-judgment way of eating that brings presence to your experience, rather than just concentrating on calories and fat intake. This mindset will help prevent you from overeating, which can get in the way of your goals and also cause indigestion. When breaking your fast, you want to ease into it with a light breakfast. Later in the morning, you could have a green smoothie or nuts, and then a regular lunch at noon. Lunch should be your biggest meal — one that is full of prebiotics — between the hours of 12 and 4 p.m., preferably closer to noon, when your digestion is really peaking. And hydrate, hydrate, hydrate — about 2.25 litres a day.

Just because you *can* eat doesn't mean you *should* eat whatever you want. Keep these tips in mind:

- Avoid refined sugars and processed carbohydrates (sugar will cause your insulin to spike).
- Moderate your protein intake — don't eat it in excess.
- Eat more natural fats, like avocados, nuts, and chia seeds.
- Eat whole, unprocessed foods.
- Stay hydrated — shoot for 2.25 litres of water a day (not including tea).

A typical week could look like the following, based on your familiarity with intermittent fasting:

Level 1 (beginner): Fast 12 hours a day 6 days a week to get your body used to the program. After 2–3 weeks, if you want, go to Level 2.

Level 2 (intermediate): Fast 4 days a week for 12 hours, and fast 2 "push" days for 15–16+ hours, with 1 day off. Do this for as long as you like.

Level 3 (advanced): Once you master the plan and want to up your game, you can add one 24-hour fast that goes from dinner to dinner — once a month. You could also stretch your push days to 18 hours from 15. But listen to your body.

This is supposed to be good for you — going too hard will just upend your progress.

❧

The following plan gives you a bird's-eye view of the Level 2 fasting plan.

- *Monday, Tuesday, Thursday, Friday* (4 days a week): Fast for 12 hours starting at or before 8 p.m.
- *Wednesday, Sunday* (2 days a week): Take an extended fast — what I call "push" days — of 15+ hours — starting around 6 p.m., ending at around 9 a.m. On these days, do some light exercise (yoga or walking).
- *Saturday* (1 day a week): Free day! No restrictions — you can eat off plan and eat at any time.

Getting into the Right Mindset

Without the right mindset, you may start out strong but will fizzle out before the two weeks are over. Like anything, you are fueled by enthusiasm in the beginning, but soon the pitfalls will start and you might want to go back to your old inflammatory ways!

The hard truth is that when you decide you are going to take care of your health and your body, it's not always an easy way forward. People may judge your decisions or question your program or, worse, make fun of you. Some days will be tough and cravings will creep up. This, unfortunately, is a fact. Your mindset should have three essential components: strong motivation, an abundant mindset, and a calm mindset. With those three components, you will be able to navigate these inevitable hurdles.

What's Your Motivation?

First, think about your motivation to becoming healthier, the "why" behind your decision: Is it so you have more energy

---

for your kids? To be a good role model for your coworkers or patients? Improving your health, preventing disease, or just always becoming a better version of yourself? Remembering your motivation will help during difficult times in your journey. I recommend writing out your reasons for this change in lifestyle and putting it somewhere that you'll see regularly, as a reminder—your bathroom mirror is a good option for most.

Now, keeping your "why" in mind, imagine the likely hurdles and pitfalls you'll face along your journey. How will you handle it when you go out to dinner with your parents and they insist you eat things that don't make you feel good? What will you say? What will you do? How will you overcome those stressful situations, where it seems nothing but sugary processed food can soothe you? It's important to prepare for these situations and to always, always have your motivation front and center at these times.

Creating a Mindset of Abundance

Once you have picked your motivation, you need to tap into an abundance mindset, which means that everything is plentiful —time, money, love. Don't rush; remember, you have so much potential, opportunities are all around. If your friend succeeds —applaud him or her. Just because someone succeeds does not mean you won't. It's just like the saying: a high tide raises all boats! This mindset will help you harness calm when you start worrying or getting stressed.

I also recommend checking out Michael Hyatt, who has a podcast and has written articles that can help you get into this mindset of abundance. I listened to him when I was first trying to reset mine. The website Mindbodygreen.com has wonderful classes specifically designed to help you cultivate abundance. I also recommend David Goggins's book *Can't Hurt Me* (a game changer for me), Jen Sincero's *You Are a Badass*, and really anything by Stephen Covey, Deepak Chopra, and Tim Ferriss. There are tons of great voices out there—find someone who speaks to you.

Build That Mental Brick House

The last component of a great mindset is inner calm. Inner

calm is the feeling you harness when the world around you is in chaos. You cannot change the external world, but you can change your internal world. If you can start to practice cultivating inner calm twice a day, you will have great success in this plan. You will make better decisions, and you will be more present. Here's how to practice calm:

1. Start with a simple, quick meditation: Take three long deep breaths — six counts in, and six counts out. Try not to think about anything but the breath going in and then going out.
2. Do this breathing mini meditation three times a day.
3. When something bad happens, tell yourself that you are not going to let someone rob you of your calm, and breathe again.
4. Do at least five yoga stretches — moving and stretching your tight muscles can really help get you into your calm state. The five I do are a standing stretch, then a standing forward fold, a seated twist, a backbend, and then a seated forward fold. Forward folds are especially helpful when not in a yoga studio.
5. Think to yourself when you start to get rushed: *I have plenty of time, there is so much time* — this will give you the calm to do your task without being rushed. It's actually faster that way!
6. When you get angry, repeat this mantra: *I am peaceful, I am happy. I won't let anyone change that.*
7. Get plenty of sleep — 8+ hours have been shown to increase calming hormones.

Commit to doing at least two of the above practices every day for the rest of this plan. If you do this in a calm, methodical way, you are destined for success.

WHEN TO STOP FASTING

If you notice any of the negative hormonal imbalance symptoms I mentioned, if you experience problems with your menstrual cycles, or if fasting triggers symptoms of an eating disorder, then stop immediately.

How to Sync IF with Your Menstrual Cycle

It's important to sync exercise and food with your period cycle. Your period cycle begins on day one, the first day of your period, with the follicular phase, which is about 14–16 days. This is when your hormone levels are low, but as you progress through this phase, estrogen starts to rise and you become much more insulin sensitive. This leads to less fat storage, and you're more resilient to stress, meaning cortisol levels tend to be low at this time of the month. This translates into you feeling more energetic. It also means you're able to tolerate more carbohydrates and more-stressful workouts. You can also be more aggressive with your intermittent fasting.

The second half of your cycle is called the luteal phase, which is more progesterone dominant, making you less insulin sensitive (you want to be insulin sensitive). Even though this tends to make you hungry, you want to avoid too many carbohydrates, especially simple carbs (say no to chocolate or even a sweet potato). Rely more on nuts and magnesium-rich foods like avocados and dark leafy greens, especially in the last week of the luteal phase, the week right before your period. During this phase, do fewer stress-inducing activities and more stress-reducing activities like walking and yoga.

Even if you are on birth control, your cycles will follow this hormonal pattern, as the pill tries to mimic the estrogen-dominant and progesterone-dominant phases of our cycles. Either way, I recommend tracking your cycle. Bottom line: you can do intermittent fasting throughout this entire cycle, except for the week before your period, when you may want to do shorter fasting intervals (12 hours) to be a little gentler on your body and to avoid raising cortisol levels.

Optimizing Exercise and Fasting for a Woman

MENSTRUAL CYCLE

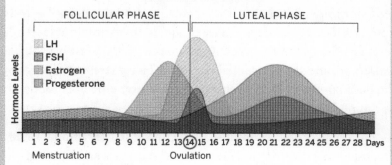

FOLLICULAR PHASE — LUTEAL PHASE

- LH
- FSH
- Estrogen
- Progesterone

Hormone Levels

1 2 3 4 5 6 7 8 9 10 11 12 13 (14) 15 16 17 18 19 20 21 22 23 24 25 26 27 28 Days

Menstruation — Ovulation

WEEKS OF THE MENSTRUAL CYCLE

Weeks 1 & 2:
FAST AGGRESSIVELY AND WORK OUT AGGRESSIVELY.

Week 4 (Before Period):
Increase stress-reducing activities like walking and yoga and decrease carbohydrate consumption.
NO or VERY EASY fasting.
(Note: Week 3 is a hybrid of weeks 2 and 4.)

	30	31	1	2	3	4	5
Week 1	(6)	7	8	9	10	11	12
Week 2	(13)	14	15	16	17	18	19
Week 3	20	21	22	23	24	25	26
Week 4	(27)	28	29	30	31	1	2

PHASES OF THE MENSTRUAL CYCLE

Follicular Phase (Days 0–14):
The follicular phase is a time when follicles grow and prepare for ovulation. Eat more healthy carbs like sweet potatoes, fruits, and oats. You are more insulin sensitive.

Luteal Phase (Days 15–28):
You are more insulin resistant, so eat more vegetables, seeds, and nuts and less sugar or carbohydrates.

THE BASICS OF THE FAST

The key to fasting effectively is to do it at an interval that makes sense for *you* — one that you will actually maintain. I do a 14- to 16-hour fast about three days in a week, and try to maintain at least a 12-hour fast the rest of the week. Outside of circadian fasting, the plan centers around three essential parts that I have stressed throughout the book: 6–8 servings of vegetables daily, prebiotic fiber foods, and hormone-balancing tea.

- *Eat Your Vegetables:* Because of the decreased nutritional value and loss of diversity in grains, they should be a small part of our diet. We need to really increase the amount of vegetables — local organic is best — to amounts most Americans do not get: 6–8 servings. Vegetables contain hundreds to thousands of phytonutrients — literally plant hormones — that have a hormone-balancing effect in the body. Vegetables (as well as fruit) also supply us with fiber that binds itself to old estrogen, thereby clearing it out of the system, leading to better overall equilibrium. This is great for both men and women who suffer from estrogen dominance.
- *Eat Prebiotic Fiber:* Most Americans get 10–15 grams of fiber a day, much less than the 25 grams needed for a woman and 35 grams for a man. Fiber is sorely needed for good gut bacteria to grow. Vegetables are the perfect type of prebiotics — fiber-rich foods that feed the good bacteria. Eating these prebiotic foods at every meal is key to strengthen the gut-immune-hormone connection. Think asparagus, artichoke, leafy greens, garlic, onion, and chicory root. Typically, you should have two large vegetable-based meals a day.
- *Drink Hormone-Balancing Tea:* Around the world, more than coffee, tea is the most frequently ingested liquid after water. There have been recent studies confirming the benefits of tea, including its hormone-balancing, anti-carcinogenic, anti-adhesive, antibacterial, and possible prebiotic effects. The benefits of tea — any kind of tea, really — are even greater than

coffee, and it has fewer side effects than other anti-inflammatory drinks like wine. Speaking of coffee, avoid all-day caffeine. One to three cups a day is okay for those who can tolerate it, but excessive caffeine raises your cortisol and slows down your thyroid. (Check out my Go-to Hormone-Balancing Chai Latte recipe on page 224; you can make it decaf or full throttle.) Alcohol is okay in small amounts. In my research, it has been repeatedly shown to be beneficial for gut hormones and energy. However, it has to be in the right amounts — and quality matters. If you choose to drink, limit your consumption to one glass during the eating period.

- *Watch Your Protein:* To me, having too much protein in a diet is just as bad as having too much sugar. This turns off the autophagy, which helps us restore and repair our bodies. Many cancer studies show dietary protein as a factor. Be careful with high-protein diets — a lot of protein can wreak havoc on our systems. You can get adequate protein much easier than you think — you don't need the bars, the protein powders, and muscle milk. While I personally stay away from red meat, one daily serving of fresh fish or grass-fed meat like chicken is okay.

Meat Eater?

I grew up as a vegetarian — so following a mainly plant-based plan was not such a transition for me. Still, I struggled to give up the dairy in my chai tea and really feel empathetic to people who struggle transitioning to a plant-based diet. My point: don't feel like you need to be 100 percent vegan or even vegetarian. Eating a wide variety of plants is key to getting fiber and phytonutrients. You can have a junk-food vegan or vegetarian diet (believe me, I grew up in a household where we ate a ton of junk carbohydrates and sugar even though we didn't eat any animal products). This plan is all about making meaningful and healthy changes that you can build on over time – start by limiting meat and animal products to once a day and adding in more plants, and you can choose to go more plant-based from there, if desired.

TWO-WEEK CIRCADIAN FASTING

Ready to start your path to wellness? Over the next two weeks, you will do varying lengths of fasts, building up to the long fasts of 15–18 hours. The more you fast, the easier it gets . . . I promise. Please remember these are *guidelines* — if you need to shift the hours later or earlier to structure around your schedule, please do so, as long as you are still following your circadian clock. Feel free to mix up lunch and dinner menus!

The Fast at a Glance

Week 1

Day 1	12 hours: 8 p.m. to 8 a.m.
Day 2	12 hours: 8 p.m. to 8 a.m.
Day 3	15 hours: 6 p.m. to 9 a.m.
Day 4	12 hours: 8 p.m. to 8 a.m.
Day 5	12 hours: 8 p.m. to 8 a.m.
Day 6	Free day!
Day 7	15 hours: 6 p.m. to 9 a.m.

Week 2

Day 8	12 hours: 8 p.m. to 8 a.m.
Day 9	12 hours: 8 p.m. to 8 a.m.
Day 10	15 hours: 6 p.m. to 9 a.m.
Day 11	12 hours: 8 p.m. to 8 a.m.
Day 12	12 hours: 8 p.m. to 8 a.m.
Day 13	Free day!
Day 14	16 hours: 6 p.m. to 10 a.m.

Week 1

Day 1

Okay, this is it. You ready? The plan is for you to stop eating by 8 p.m. and fast for 12 hours. Have breakfast at 8 a.m. with lunch at noon and dinner at 6 p.m. Since this is day 1, you may struggle tonight — I am here to tell you that is totally fine, and actually pretty common. If you feel hungry, drink water, but if that still does not satisfy, then find a snack that is 40 calories or less (for example, a spoonful of nut butter). Get plenty of rest tonight, and tomorrow morning make sure you get some morning sun, even if it is cold or cloudy. Your body can absorb some vitamin D from the UV rays poking through the clouds, so try to get outside and walk for about 20 minutes.

Breakfast at 8 a.m.: Almond-Vanilla Chia Seed Pudding (see recipe, page 224)

Snack at 10 a.m.

Lunch at noon: Green Gut Smoothie (see recipe, page 230) plus veggies and hummus

Dinner at 6 p.m.: Eggplant "Parm" (see recipe, page 254)

Snack at 7 p.m.

Snacks While Fasting

Just because you are lowering inflammation does not mean that you cannot have treats once in a while! If you get hungry during your fasting period, try to curb your hunger with water or non-caloric drinks like coffee or tea (in the morning, to avoid having caffeine too late in the day). If the hunger does not dissipate, then eat something that is 40 calories or less, such as

- ½ tablespoon of nut butter
- Thin slice of avocado

- Cup of herbal tea with a splash of almond milk
- Glass of homemade lemonade with stevia (I liked to spice up mine with a pinch of cayenne pepper)

I try to stay away from any type of sugar, period, and in particular while fasting, but a little bit of stevia is okay as long as whatever you have is within the 40-calorie mark.

Snacks During the Eating Window
Of course, do not overindulge — one serving of snacks in a day should be plenty if you are eating enough at meals. Here are the snacks and treats to have when you are in your eating window (not while fasting).

- 10–15 dark chocolate chips
- 75 g of nuts
- 125 g hummus and carrots
- Homemade smoothies (see recipes, pages 226, 230)
- 2 tablespoons of peanut butter with celery
- 150 g air-popped popcorn, with some non-GMO olive oil
- 100 g fresh berries or watermelon
- 50–75 g anti-inflammatory trail mix: blend equal amounts of coconut flakes, raw nuts, and dried goji berries
- Chia seed pudding (see recipes, pages 224, 225)

Day 2
You successfully made it through your first fast, so give yourself a pat on the back.

Tonight starts another 12-hour fast; here's the breakdown:

Breakfast at 8 a.m.: Orange-Cardamom Chia Seed Pudding (see recipe, page 225)

Snack at 10 a.m.

Lunch at noon: Healthy Gut Salad (see recipe, page 232)

Dinner at 6 p.m.: Creamy Cauliflower Soup
(see recipe, page 236)

Snack at 7 p.m.

Day 3

This is it—the first "push" day of a fast for 15 hours, your longest fast so far. Remember, if you are new to intermittent fasting, you can modify (12 hours is the minimum) and then work up from there. If you are hungry and it does not pass in 30 minutes, have a spoonful of almond butter or a few slices of avocado. A little fat is the key to tiding over the hunger until it's time to break the fast.

Breakfast at 8 a.m.: Chocolate Green Shake
(see recipe, page 231)

Snack at 10 a.m.

Lunch at noon: Healthy Gut Salad (see recipe, page 232)

Snack at 3 p.m.

Note: Go a bit higher in calories for lunch, and remember to eat fiber in addition to a protein that will sustain you until dinner. I often combine tofu with a salad that has a lot of beans and chickpeas. A dairy or nondairy yogurt could be a great supplement to this meal.

Dinner at 5:30 p.m.: Healthy Nachos (see recipe, page 246)

Fast starting at 6 p.m. until 9 a.m. the next morning.

Day 4

You made it through the longest fast of the program! For those of you who modified the fasting time, you can build up to the 15-hour fast through the remaining duration of the program. The fast tonight should be relatively easy. You should be finding the fast a bit easier by now and, if all goes well, really start feeling better. You are back to doing a 12-hour fast today.

Breakfast at 9 a.m.: Orange-Cardamom Chia Seed Pudding (see recipe, page 225)

Lunch at noon: Healthy Gut Salad (see recipe, page 232)

Snack at 3 p.m.

Dinner at 6 p.m.: One-Pan Roasted Asparagus and Brussels Sprouts (see recipe, page 248)

Snack at 7 p.m.

Day 5

Today is another 12-hour fast. Have dinner at 6 p.m., then a snack around 7 p.m., and your fast begins at 8 p.m. You will break your fast in the morning at 8 a.m.

Breakfast at 8 a.m.: Chocolate Green Shake (see recipe, page 231)

Snack at 10 a.m.

Lunch at noon: Healthy Gut Salad (see recipe, page 232)

Dinner at 6 p.m.: Penne "Alfredo" with Roasted Cauliflower (see recipe, page 256)

Snack at 7 p.m.

Day 6

You deserve a free day! This is the time to enjoy a meal with your loved ones at a restaurant or eat some of the foods you really enjoy. Whatever it is, make sure you are not keeping an unhealthy addiction alive. Try to make smart and healthy choices. Try to minimize your fat and sugar intake, eat plenty of protein and vegetables, get your fiber, and stay hydrated.

Day 7

Today's fast is another "push" day. Dinner is at 5:30 p.m., and then stop eating by 6 p.m. You can break your fast at 9 a.m. the next morning.

Breakfast at 8 a.m.: Orange-Cardamom Chia Seed Pudding (see recipe, page 225)

Snack at 10 a.m.

Lunch at noon: Healthy Gut Salad (see recipe, page 232)

Snack at 3 p.m.

Dinner at 5:30 p.m.: Sweet Potato–Crust Veggie Pizza (see recipe, page 251)

Stop eating by 6 p.m. and fast until 9 a.m. the next morning.

Week 2

Halfway there! Quick tip: Stop eating when you are 50 percent full and walk away from your food for at least 15 minutes. Drink water or tea or brush your teeth. You'll start to recognize the feeling of being satisfied and light, not full.

Day 8

Rinse and repeat of last week — you can do it. Remember to drink plenty of water and have a 40-calorie or less snack while fasting, if needed. Please remember to minimize your exercise after 6 p.m. The most you should do is go for a walk. You can't beat fresh air.

Breakfast at 9 a.m.: Almond-Vanilla Chia Seed Pudding (see recipe, page 224)

Lunch at noon: Green Gut Smoothie (see recipe, page 230) and veggies and hummus

Snack at 3 p.m.

Dinner at 6 p.m.: Falafel Salad with Tahini Dressing (see recipe, page 235)

Snack at 7 p.m.

Day 9

Today's schedule is a fast from 8 p.m. to 8 a.m. the next day. Easy peasy.

Breakfast at 8 a.m.: Orange-Cardamom Chia Seed Pudding (see recipe, page 225)

Snack at 10 a.m.

Lunch at noon: Healthy Gut Salad (see recipe, page 232)

Dinner at 6 p.m.: Vegetable-Oats Dosa (see recipe, page 269)

Snack at 7 p.m.

Day 10

Push day, 15 hours. You got this.

Breakfast at 8 a.m.: Tea with a handful of nuts

Snack at 10 a.m.: Chocolate Green Shake (see recipe, page 231)

Lunch at noon: Healthy Gut Salad (see recipe, page 232)

Dinner at 5:30 p.m.: Simple Indian-Spiced Chickpeas (see recipe, page 250)

Stop eating by 6 p.m. and fast until 9 a.m. the next morning.

A Typical Amy Shah Fasting Day

Breakfast, 8 a.m.: Today, after getting my sunshine to solidify my circadian clock, I ate a bowl of berries and drank an oat milk latte with stevia to break my fast from the previous day. I also had a shake with a half-scoop vegan protein chocolate powder, almond milk, ice, and stevia. (As you know, I do not like to add too much artificial protein, but it's okay once in a while in a pinch.)

Morning snack, 10 a.m.: I had a bag of pistachios and a kombucha drink — kombucha has an added probiotic benefit and has a bit of sweetness to curb those sugar urges.

Lunch, noon: This is an important meal because the combined calories of lunch and dinner have to get you through your long fast. Today I had a big bowl of lentil dal, nondairy yogurt, and Indian-style sweet potatoes and spinach that I packed in my lunch bag.

Dinner, 5:30 p.m.: For dinner tonight, Mexican. I had a black bean bowl with a whole avocado and pico de gallo over cauliflower rice. I added fresh salsa as a tasty topping. I treated myself to a handful of keto chocolate chips for dessert with a few added pieces of dark chocolate!

Day 11

Today is an easy day with a 12-hour fast.

Breakfast at 9 a.m.: Almond-Vanilla Chia Seed Pudding (see recipe, page 224)

Lunch at noon: Healthy Gut Salad (see recipe, page 232)

Snack at 3 p.m.

Dinner at 6 p.m.: Grilled Balsamic Portobello Mushrooms with Sun-Dried Tomato-Basil "Mayo" (see recipe, page 248)

Snack at 7 p.m.

Day 12

As we head into the last few days of the program, I would like for you to try to do your best to stick with the schedule for the next three days. Let's end the program on a high note.

Breakfast at 8 a.m.: Chocolate Green Shake
(see recipe, page 231)

Snack at 10 a.m.

Lunch at 12 p.m.: Healthy Gut Salad (see recipe, page 232)

Dinner at 6 p.m.: Black Bean Burgers (see recipe, page 253)

Snack at 7 p.m.

Note: Keep in mind, it is okay to occasionally adjust the fasting schedule to better suit your own schedule, especially on weekends. For example, if there's a party on Friday night, then you can push back the starting time by one hour and end your fast Saturday morning one hour later. Or if you have a work dinner one night, you can adjust your breakfast time the next day accordingly. Sometimes we need to make changes to make things work with our own life. The purpose of intermittent fasting is to get your whole body healthy again, so make it work for you. If you stress about the schedule, then you are partially negating what you are trying to do. Stress increases your cortisol, which can lead to overeating and cause your body to store fat.

Day 13

Free day!

Day 14

Your last push day. No problem, right?!

Breakfast at 8 a.m.: Orange-Cardamom Chia Seed Pudding (see recipe, page 225)

Snack at 10 a.m.

Lunch at noon: Healthy Gut Salad (see recipe, page 232)

Dinner at 5:30 p.m.: Quick Vegan Pho (see recipe, page 264)

Stop eating by 6 p.m. and fast until 10 a.m. the next morning.

The biggest thing is to plan how you will break your fast. As usual, I will likely break with a chai, green juice, a cup of raw nuts, berries, and raw veggies with hummus. If you feel like that's a lot of chewing (LOL), a smoothie with all of these ingredients works well.

❧

You made it through two weeks of fasting! How do you feel? I hope you loved the results it gave you, so much so that you continue intermittent fasting on a more regular basis. If you fast sporadically, remember that your gut deserves and needs a rest. Let your body and mind reset from time to time — you will be surprised how impactful a short break can be both physically and mentally. I hope you incorporate some of these principles into your health and wellness journey. Tomorrow morning you can break your fast at any time since the program is officially over. If you can, try to go the 12 hours tonight, since it should be fairly easy for you to do so by now.

Made it this far? Congrats! You feel good? I hope so! What should you do now — just go back to your regular life? No! This is a marathon, not a sprint. Most studies show and most patients I work with notice the most improvement over one to two years' time — the longer you do this, the more you'll see results. Give yourself a chance to heal and change, and you will feel results that will last a lifetime.

Nature Does the Body Good

We are living in a modern world that is more removed from nature than ever: we are stuck indoors glued to our TVs or computer screens; we drive in our air-conditioned cars to our temperature-controlled offices with stark fluorescent lighting. But research shows that we need nature more than ever. Exhaustive studies underscore the importance of spending time outside, which has significant and wide-ranging health benefits, including reducing the risk of type 2 diabetes, cardiovascular disease, and high blood pressure and lowering mortality rates.

Besides all that, think of all that time you are away from your computer, phone, and social media — unplugging outside is one of the best things you can do for your stress levels. Some studies also show how nature can benefit your productivity. In 2015 the *Journal of Environmental Psychology* noted a phenomenon called "biophilia," which is our innate desire to be connected with nature, and showed how taking a "micro-break" to view a green — not concrete — city scene sustained attention and gave a sense of relaxation. The study group who had a green scene performed significantly better and made fewer mistakes than those who had a city rooftop scene.[5] This shows us that even if you can't get yourself to a forest or beach, *just viewing* images of nature can provide positive effects.

Here are some ways you can work nature into your everyday routine:

- Get barefoot. Go out to your backyard, front lawn, or a park, take off your shoes, and walk around for a little while. Of course don't go walking around in grass treated with chemicals or that may be full of ticks, but no matter where you live, there should be some patch of earth outside you can tickle your toes with.
- Take a walk on the beach! Can you think of anything more grounding than walking in the sand, watching the waves crash in, and breathing in salt air?

- Have a picnic on a lawn. Sit on a blanket alone or with company and put your feet in the grass, have a meal, play cards, or just get lost in conversation.
- Take a yoga class outside and stand in mountain pose with your toes in the dirt.
- Take a hike in the canyons, the mountains, or a nature preserve. Go somewhere far away from the clatter of cars and the energy of modern life.
- Swim in a lake or ocean.
- Climb a tree; read a book leaning your back against the trunk; play in the leaves.
- Visit a farm or agricultural center. Touch stuff. Go apple picking.
- Run your hands in the dirt; hold some soil in your hands; make some mud.

Even if you roll down your window while you drive on your way to work for just a few minutes, I promise you will get a quick jolt of clarity and focus.

ALL THE RIGHT MOVES

I remember how exhilarated I used to feel after an hours-long run (yes, I said *hours*). The sheer exhaustion, the sore legs, the achy joints . . . I thought, *This means I'm doing something good for my body.* But in my sweat-drenched bliss, I had no idea that those long cardio sessions were doing serious damage. As it turns out, more is not better when it comes to cardio. In fact, too much of it — like too much of anything — can slowly kill you.

I can already hear you asking, "But I thought cardio was good for the heart?" And more is better, right? Not always. Research among people who run marathons, ultra-marathons, Ironman-length triathlons, and participate in other endurance sports suggests chronic cardio can cause heart dysfunction, plaque buildup, and stiff arteries. Another study found something similar: Just after a race, some endurance runners had troubling cardiac problems, including a weakened right ventricle. Most recovered within a week of the race, but some of these elite runners had existing heart damage despite (or, perhaps, because of) all that cardio.

What does that mean for the rest of us non-elite athletes? At the very least, it throws a serious wrench in this idea that the best exercise is both intense and sustained. A recent study suggests that slower joggers live longer than strenuous ones. Chronic cardio can send your hormones into a tailspin, particularly when it comes to cortisol. This stress hormone is okay in small doses, but when you have too much, it can be one of the most potent saboteurs to your health.

ENERGY BOOSTER

A fasted workout—exercising before you break your fast in the morning—is hugely beneficial because you are optimizing autophagy in three ways: One, you are extending your fast, and hence extending autophagy as well. Two, by working out, you are ramping up the rate of autophagy working in your body. Three, you turn on that metabolic switch mode—when we deplete our glycogen stores and we switch our fuel sources to fat-burning ketones—that is so good for us. Plus, if you exercise outdoors, you can optimize your circadian rhythm by taking in natural sunlight before 10 a.m. It's a wonderful cocktail of anti-aging regimens all in one before you really start your day!

When you do too much cardio, your body generates soaring levels of cortisol. Producing too much instructs your brain to store fat (especially around your abdomen) and inhibits your body's ability to process sugar. If sugar isn't processed properly, you gain weight.

So, what do you do instead?

Try yoga along with nature walks and hikes interspersed with cardio.

Yoga is a mind-body exercise that's sometimes a hard transition for cardio lovers. But it's likely worth incorporating if you're busy, have higher stress, and want to transform your mindset.

It turns out that yoga practice is as good — if not better — for your health as other types of exercise, particularly when it comes to taking it easy on your body's stress system (i.e., cortisol). Yoga has also been found to lower blood pressure, increase flexibility, decrease persistent pain, and improve posture, to name a few benefits.

Not a fan of yoga or need something that's quick? Try high-intensity interval training, otherwise known as HIIT. A HIIT workout is less about sustained effort and more about doing your exercise in fits and starts. Start your workout with a 1- to 2- minute warm-up, followed by a 30-second sprint. For me, that means an all-out run or, if I'm on a treadmill, running up an incline of about 9.5 percent. Follow it up with a 1-minute cool-down, followed by another 30-second sprint. Do this for 8 minutes, every other day, and I guarantee you'll notice a change in two weeks. The other benefits? It's something studies increasingly say is good for your heart. Is this convincing enough to finally give up on running marathons? It was for me!

No matter what you pick, all I ask is that you move for 20 minutes a day — preferably in sunlight. Be mindful of the type of exercise you integrate into your daily routine. Limit CrossFit or high-intensity training to three times a week, and on the remaining days opt for low-intensity exercises such as walking 8,000–12,000 steps a day and practicing yoga. Being easy on your body is best when trying to regulate any type of hormonal imbalance.

Remember to do the workouts to make the most of your fitness routine and gut rest. When you are doing the extended fasts, don't do long (> 60 minutes), hard workouts. Stick to yoga or a short HIIT session.

Beautiful on the Inside and on the Outside

Remember that it's not just what you put in your body that is important; it is what you put on it, too: Skip the perfume and any paraben-containing cosmetics. Skip or switch your deodorant to a natural one like Tom's of Maine. Unless it's super-hot, you do not need to use a deodorant on a daily basis — it can actually kill the good bacteria of your armpits and foster the bad (and smelly) bacteria.

Every week or two, try to get rid of one more thing that can be toxic. It's difficult but doable. To be honest, this has been by far the hardest part of my transformation, so I started with one product swap-out every few weeks. Again, use baby steps — start by avoiding eating and drinking from plastic and by using natural cleansers and soaps.

ENERGY BOOSTER

There's so much information on the health benefits of saunas. Saunas are also considered a hormetic stressor and are known to improve the cardiovascular system, aid in post-workout recovery, get rid of toxins, bolster the immune system, help with sleep, cleanse the skin, and relieve stress. There is a risk of dehydration, so I suggest keeping sauna time from 15 to 20 minutes. And while I recommend saunas, heated exercise is even better. Find a hot yoga or HIIT class, and get that glorious glow!

Supplements

Work with a practitioner to figure out the combination that is right for you, but here are ones I commonly recommend:

vitamin D, omega-3, maca root, turmeric, rhodiola, and vitamins B_6, B_9, and B_{12}. But remember, work with your doctor and personalize to your needs. Take supplements in addition to eating well, sleeping, and exercise for greater impact, but no supplement ever trumps a good diet, fasting, exercise, and self-care.

ENERGY BUSTER

There is a lot of research on how intermittent fasting may impact women's reproductive cycles and reproductive health. With this in mind, take a cautious approach to intermittent fasting if you have never fasted before. Talk to your doctor before beginning the program, and know your body and its nutrient needs. Definitely do not start intermittent fasting if you are pregnant, lactating, or plan to get pregnant.

Be Social

According to Harvard's Grant and Glueck Study, which tracked hundreds of participants over the course of 75 years, our relationships have a huge impact on our health. Robert Waldinger, the Harvard study's director, says: "The clearest message that we get from this 75-year study is this: Good relationships keep us happier and healthier. Period."[6] In other words, the company we keep is key to long-term happiness and fulfillment. Weed out toxic friends; keep the ones who lift you up. And keep in touch often.

Reduce Stress

When you wake up, be present. Take a moment to focus on an action or a sensation. For example, as you walk, focus on each step and the sensations you feel as each foot touches the ground and lifts back off, or notice what the chair underneath you feels like. Giving yourself this awareness and pause is a great stress reducer you can do anywhere, anytime.

In the morning — ideally before breakfast — get on a yoga mat. Studies indicate that yoga decreases inflammation.[7] Besides the obvious mindfulness and breathing aspects of yoga, the twisting, strengthening, and stretching poses have been shown to reduce biological markers of inflammation and detoxify and balance the body systemically. If you are not sure how to get started, check out some online beginner programs; I personally like Yoga with Adriene, Gaia, and Strala Yoga. For in-person classes, check out your local yoga studios and find one that will fit your needs.

Halfway through your day, do a few deep breathing exercises. Deep breathing exercises build strength and resilience in the body, greatly reducing stress and, therefore, inflammation. They also slow the mind and central nervous system, allowing the body to relax deeply.

If you can swing it, getting a massage is a twofold strategy to reduce physical and emotional stress. Getting touched has been indicated to decrease anxiety, lower blood pressure, increase serotonin, and help with sleep.[8]

Massage stimulates lymph flow, pumping oxygen and nutrients into tissues and vital organs, improving circulation and immunity. It is not only deliciously relaxing mentally and physiologically, but it also softens and repairs injured, tired, and overused (inflamed) muscles and tissue. Do I have to tell you twice to get a massage?

I also recommend cultivating a meditation practice. Daily meditation changes neurological pathways that make us more resilient to stress. There are many ways to meditate, from Transcendental Meditation that uses a mantra, to guided meditation, to chanting or simply just sitting still for a few minutes. There's a meditation practice for everyone. There are so many apps that can get you started, like Headspace, Calm, and Aura. Find one that suits you and work it into your lifestyle.

Finally, two hours before bed, turn off your devices. The constant beeping, messaging, and rapid-fire stimulation of our phones, computers, and televisions create anxiety, overstimulation, and stress. Have periods when you turn them all off. Talk to someone, take a walk, play a game, or listen to music and dance. Yes, dancing reduces inflammation — so put on some Prince or Taylor Swift or whoever gets your booty shaking.

THE FOREVER PLAN

Congrats, you've made it through the two-week WTF plan! I hope you love your results so much that you would like to implement this in the long term — what I like to call the forever plan. But first, ask yourself these questions:

- How do you feel?
- Was the program hard to do? Did you love it or hate it?
- How tired do you feel in the morning when you wake up?
- How tired are you in the afternoon?
- Are you able to put more energy into your workouts?
- How much do you suffer bloating or cravings?

Chances are in just two weeks you have seen positive changes to your energy levels, your mood, and your gut. While we know that the GI tract can change its epithelium (the gut lining) within five to seven days, getting used to a new routine takes longer. So it's not that the GI tract needs more time, it's that YOU need more time to create a habit that can generate benefits to last your entire life. More important, studies show that doing intermittent fasting long term is really when you'll start to see major changes in your health markers: cholesterol, blood pressure, C-reactive protein (an inflammation marker), and weight all go down. And, really, these incredible changes don't happen so early in the diet.

❧

This two-week plan could just be the beginning for you on the road to full energy restoration. So I say continue on the journey. Continue the plan for three months, which is just about the right amount of time needed to make something automatic. Then, after those three months, check in with your progress. If you like what you see and how you feel, do it for another three months. And another and another . . . rinse and repeat . . . forever.

A three-month forever plan looks like this:

6 days of fasting: depending on your lifestyle and experience, fast between 12 and 18 hours for 4–5 days, with 2–3 push days of 16–18 fasting hours.
1 day completely off

Exceptions to the Rule

Look, I know life is filled with social engagements, work dinners, birthdays, and holidays. These can be minefields for some people who are trying to eat right, but if you know what to do ahead of time, you can get through them without sabotaging your plan. There are easy modifications that will help you stay on track (the same can't be said of avoiding talking to your crazy uncle during the holidays).

Option 1: Try to stick to your schedule of fasting 12–16 hours and time restrict on a big meal by starting to eat by 3 p.m. and stopping at around 6 or 7 p.m., then give yourself a long fasting window until about 9 or 10 a.m. the next morning. (This is perfect for an otherwise gluttonous Thanksgiving.)

Option 2: Calorie restrict. During a holiday season or summer vacation, it may be hard to miss those fun late dinners. Calorie restriction, limiting your caloric intake — about 25 percent less than your usual intake — can be a good alternative. Eat until you're 75 percent full; don't stuff yourself with everything you see.

Option 3: Go all out as if it's a cheat day, then fast 18–24 hours the next day. This is pretty advanced, so I wouldn't suggest this option for beginners, nor would I suggest doing this a lot, especially within a close time frame (e.g., Christmas, then again on New Year's Eve).

Frequent Q's and A's

I travel a lot. How do I adjust the fasting on my trips?

I say when in Rome . . . One of the worst things you can do if you are traveling to a place in a different time zone is to continue to eat on your old schedule. Make every effort to acclimate as soon as possible — eat (and sleep) according to the time zone you are in.

I work late, so I tend to eat late. Can I tailor this to have my last meal later in the evening (say 8–9 p.m.)?

I always say do what is going to work best for you and your circumstances. If you can, try to stick to the windows as much as possible, and if two days you have to eat later, just adjust breaking the fast accordingly. For example, if your last meal is at 9 p.m. on a 12-hour fasting window, have breakfast at 9 a.m. the next day. Sound good?

Can you exercise in the evening once you have started your fast?

Yes, but keep it easy and light — otherwise you risk your hunger pangs keeping you up late.

What is a good food to break the fast?

Honestly, there is no perfect food to break a fast, but whatever you choose should contain vegetables (surprise, surprise!). Think of the four S's — smoothies, salad, soup, and a (tofu) scramble.

*What do you do if your partner or family members are
not on board?*

Hopefully, you can persuade them to see the benefits of IF,
but if you can't, that doesn't mean you have to bag the plan for
yourself. Just eat during your designated fasting window and
when others eat later, sit with them and enjoy a cup of tea.

*OMG, I ate a cracker (oops, I mean a cookie) during my fast!
What do I do?*

If you eat a cookie, it's no big deal. Remember, this is
not about perfection. This is just about improving your
metabolism. Move on, and don't beat yourself up! Keep going
with the fast—you'll still get metabolic benefits even though
you're not completely in the fasting state.

9

The WTF Meals

NOW, HERE'S THE FUN PART — delicious food! Here are my favorite anti-inflammatory, plant-based meals that will get you on your way to having more energy. Many of the recipes that follow are healthier versions of popular recipes from around the world, handpicked and tried by me to make your health journey SIMPLE and easy. A few tips to remember:

- Try to cluster most of your calories from 12 p.m. to 5 p.m. Try not to eat within 3–4 hours of bedtime, and do not overeat during your eating window. Plan your meals in advance and eating times in advance also.
- Nutrient-dense foods are the best thing to consume while in your eating window. Translation: nuts, seeds, fruits (berries), vegetables, lean protein (sprouted tofu), whole grains, and beans. Focus on eating high-fiber, unprocessed, whole foods with lots of good-for-you herbs and spices for extra flavor.
- Try to stay away from processed and hyper-palatable foods (goodbye, Doritos and Magnolia cupcakes). Avoid meat as

much as possible, especially red meat, as well as sugar, trans fats, and refined starches.

- If you get hungry during your fasting period, try to curb your hunger with water or non-caloric drinks (coffee, tea ...). If the hunger does not dissipate, then eat something without sugar that is around 40 calories (see suggestions on page 197).
- If you are on a sugar-free diet, you can substitute raw stevia for honey or agave.
- If you are a vegan and need an egg substitute, try Bob's Red Mill Egg Replacer.
- If you are on a dairy-free diet, feel free to use any nut milk you prefer.

GROCERY LIST

The lists below are based on the meal plans I suggest in chapter 8, but please feel free to mix it up with any of the recipes in this book or any of your favorite go-to healthy meals. Remember to add to the list any teas that you like and any snacks and food for your free day.

Week 1

PANTRY

    Apple cider vinegar
    Black beans
    Cocoa powder, unsweetened
    Coconut, shredded and unsweetened
    Coconut flour
    Coconut oil
    Flaxseed oil
    All-purpose flour
    Ghee
    Honey (or agave or raw stevia)
    Marinara sauce (no sugar added)
    1 Mexican seasoning blend packet (such as Trader Joe's)

Nutritional yeast
Extra-virgin olive oil
Extra-virgin olive oil cooking spray
Penne, gluten-free or whole grain
Stone-ground corn tortilla chips
Vanilla extract
Vanilla protein powder
Vegetable broth
Optional: tofu beans and chickpeas

NUTS AND SEEDS
Chia seeds
Hemp seeds
Pecans
Optional: chopped toasted pistachios, almonds, or walnuts

FRUITS AND VEGETABLES
3–4 Granny Smith apples
1 bunch thin asparagus
2 bananas
250 g brussels sprouts
1 (1 kg) butternut squash
3 heads cauliflower
1 bunch celery
1 small cucumber
1 medium eggplant
2–3 garlic heads
2–4 limes
5–6 lemons
1 green onion
1 orange
1 jalapeño pepper
1 serrano pepper
Raspberries
1 bunch romaine leaves
1 small Roma tomato

baby spinach or baby kale
Optional: extra veggies for hummus; oranges and berries

FROZEN
Corn kernels

DAIRY
2 eggs or equivalent gluten-free vegan egg replacer
40 g shredded nondairy cheese (cheddar or pepper jack)
3.75 litres unsweetened nondairy milk (almond, soy)
1 (200 g) package shredded nondairy mozzarella
1 (500 g) whole-milk yogurt or nondairy yogurt

CONDIMENTS
Guacamole
Hummus
Fresh salsa

HERBS AND SPICES
1 bunch fresh basil
Ground cardamom
Cayenne pepper
1 bunch fresh coriander or parsley leaves
Garlic powder
Fresh ginger
Mustard seeds
Onion powder
Dried oregano
Ground black pepper
Crushed red pepper
Sea salt
Fresh thyme leaves
Fresh turmeric
Ground turmeric
Optional: fresh parsley

Week 2

PANTRY

Apple cider vinegar

Balsamic vinegar

1 (400 g) can black beans

1 litre no-chicken broth or mushroom broth

3 (400 g) cans chickpeas

Cocoa powder, unsweetened

Coconut aminos (available in major food stores)

Coconut flour

Coconut oil

Red Boat fish sauce

Flaxseed oil

Rice flour

Semolina flour

Ghee

Honey (or agave or raw stevia)

Instant oats

Quick oats

Olive oil

Sun-dried tomatoes, oil-packed

Tahini

Vanilla extract

Vanilla protein powder

Vegenaise

Bean thread vermicelli

NUTS AND SEEDS

Chopped raw almonds or walnuts

Chia seeds

Hemp seeds

Pecans

Optional: toasted pistachios

FRUITS AND VEGETABLES

1 Granny Smith apple
3 small apples
1 banana
Baby bok choy
1 bunch carrots
1 bunch celery
1 small cucumber
2 garlic heads
Kale or spinach
2 lemons
Bibb or romaine lettuce leaves
1 lime
4 portobello mushrooms
2 large shiitake mushrooms
1 green onion
1 red onion
2 small yellow onions
1 orange
2 jalapeño peppers
4 radishes
Raspberries
Mixed salad greens
2 medium tomatoes
1 zucchini
*Optional: Extra veggies to go with hummus, fresh bean sprouts,
sprig of fresh mint, extra tomato and onion, fresh berries*

DAIRY

Eggs (or equivalent gluten-free vegan egg replacer)
Unsweetened nondairy milk
Whole-milk yogurt or nondairy yogurt

CONDIMENTS

Chutney of choice
Guacamole
Hummus
Pico de gallo or salsa
Beet sauerkraut or regular sauerkraut
Optional: shredded unsweetened coconut

HERBS AND SPICES

1 bunch fresh basil
Ground cardamom
Cayenne pepper
Chili powder
1 bunch fresh coriander
Coriander
Ground cumin
Cumin seeds
1 bunch fresh dill (optional)
Garam masala
Fresh ginger
1 bunch fresh parsley leaves
Fresh ground pepper
Crushed red pepper flakes
Sea salt
Fresh turmeric or ground turmeric
Optional: star anise, stick cinnamon

Break That Fast

Breakfast is the first thing your body will use to power through your day, so make it count. I offer several recipes that I love first in the morning, but feel free to make these meals your own by swapping out your favorite fruits and spices.

Go-to Hormone-Balancing Chai Latte

Serves 2

> 480 ml water
> 2 bags unsweetened chai-spiced black tea
> ¼ teaspoon ground cardamom
> ½ teaspoon ground ginger
> 240 ml barista-style oat milk
> honey, optional
> ½ packet raw stevia
> Ground cinnamon

1. In a small saucepan, bring the water to a boil. Remove from heat and add the tea bags, cardamom, and ginger. Steep for 5 minutes.
2. Meanwhile, in another small saucepan, heat the oat milk over medium heat, whisking constantly until steaming and frothy.
3. Whisk the honey into the tea, if using. Strain tea through a very fine-mesh strainer into two mugs. Sweeten with stevia, top with the hot oat milk, and sprinkle with cinnamon.

Almond-Vanilla Chia Seed Pudding

Serves 1

> 120 ml unsweetened nondairy milk
> 60 g whole-milk yogurt or nondairy yogurt
> 2 tablespoons chia seeds
> 2 tablespoons finely chopped raw almonds or walnuts

¼ teaspoon pure vanilla extract
1 teaspoon honey or agave or ½ packet raw stevia
Optional toppings: fresh berries, shredded unsweetened
   coconut, and/or chopped toasted almonds or walnuts

1. In a small bowl, whisk together the nondairy milk, yogurt, chia seeds, raw nuts, vanilla, and honey (or other sweetener). Transfer to a small serving glass or bowl.
2. Cover and refrigerate for at least 2 hours or overnight.
3. Serve topped with fresh berries, coconut, and/or toasted nuts.

POWER PLAYER

Chia seeds may be little, but they pack a nutritional wallop with 11 grams of fiber, 4 grams of protein, and 9 grams of fat per serving. Plus they are high in calcium, magnesium, manganese, and phosphorus . . . all for the low-calorie count of 135.

Orange-Cardamom Chia Seed Pudding

Serves 1

120 ml unsweetened nondairy milk
60 g whole-milk yogurt or nondairy yogurt
2 tablespoons chia seeds
¼ teaspoon ground cardamom
½ teaspoon orange zest
1 teaspoon honey or agave or ½ packet raw stevia
Optional toppings: chopped orange sections, shredded
   unsweetened coconut, and/or chopped toasted pistachios
   or almonds

1. In a small bowl, whisk together the nondairy milk, yogurt, chia seeds, cardamom, orange zest, and honey (or other sweetener). Transfer to a small serving glass or bowl.
2. Cover and refrigerate for at least 2 hours or overnight.
3. Serve topped with chopped orange sections, coconut, and/or toasted nuts.

Prebiotic Matcha Smoothie Bowl

Serves 2

120 ml unsweetened flax milk
100 g frozen peach slices
50 g baby spinach leaves
2 teaspoons high-quality matcha powder
50 g cooked chickpeas (or use canned, rinsed and drained)
2 frozen bananas, cut into chunks
2 tablespoons ground flaxseed
Optional toppings: chia seeds, hemp hearts, fresh raspberries, and/or blueberries

1. In a high-powered blender, combine the flax milk, peaches, spinach, matcha powder, chickpeas, banana chunks, and flaxseed. Start on low speed and gradually increase the speed to high and blend until smooth. (If mixture is too thick, add a little water.)
2. Divide mixture between two bowls. Add desired toppings.

To store: Leftovers can be stored in a tightly sealed container in the freezer. Let defrost slightly before eating.

Note: Matcha is either culinary or ceremonial grade in quality, with varying degrees of quality within those two categories. Use good culinary-grade matcha — it will be a dull green (not muddy brown) — or very good ceremonial-grade matcha in this recipe. It will be a nice bright green. The very high-quality ceremonial-grade matcha is too expensive for this use, and the low-grade culinary matcha is full of stems and has a bitter flavor.

Banana Oatmeal Muffins

Makes 12 muffins

275 g plain whole-milk Greek yogurt

2 large eggs (or equivalent gluten-free vegan egg replacer prepared according to package directions)

2 tablespoons honey, agave, or raw stevia for baking

1 teaspoon pure vanilla extract

2 very ripe bananas

275 g rolled or quick oats

1½ teaspoons baking powder

½ teaspoon baking soda

¼ teaspoon ground cinnamon

¼ teaspoon fine sea salt

90 g walnut halves, coarsely chopped

1. Preheat the oven to 200°C/180°C fan. Line a standard 12-cup muffin tin with paper liners.

2. In a high-powered blender, combine the yogurt, eggs, honey (or other sweetener), vanilla, bananas, oats, baking powder, baking soda, cinnamon, and salt. (It's very important to put the liquids in the blender first. If you put the oats in first, they will simply get pulverized and will form hard lumps around the blades.) Start on low speed and gradually increase the speed to high and blend until smooth, scraping down the sides of the blender as needed, about 2 minutes. Transfer to a bowl and stir the walnuts in by hand.

3. Divide the batter among the muffin cups, filling each cup three-quarters of the way.

4. Bake for 15 minutes, or until a toothpick inserted in the center of the muffins comes out clean.

5. Let cool in the pan on a wire rack for 10 minutes, then remove from the pan. Serve warm or let cool completely.

Cocoa-Oat Prebiotic Breakfast Bars

Makes 16 bars

3 tablespoons coconut oil, melted, plus more for
   greasing the pan
250 g rolled or quick oats
25 g unsweetened cocoa powder
120 g dried unsweetened apple
100 g fresh blueberries
100 g raw almonds, chopped
50 g ground flaxseed
1 teaspoon ground cinnamon
50 g unsweetened applesauce
40 g fresh raspberries
75 g natural creamy almond butter
2 very ripe bananas
4 tablespoons honey, agave, or raw stevia for baking
½ teaspoon fine sea salt

1. Preheat the oven to 190°C/170°C fan. Grease an 28 x 18-cm
   baking pan with melted coconut oil. Set aside.
2. In a large bowl, stir together the oats, cocoa powder, apple,
   blueberries, almonds, flaxseed, and cinnamon.
3. In a high-powered blender, combine the 3 tablespoons coconut
   oil, applesauce, raspberries, almond butter, bananas, honey (or
   other sweetener), and salt. Blend until smooth.
4. Gently fold the blended fruit mixture into the oat mixture
   until all ingredients are very well incorporated. Let stand for
   15 minutes.
5. Press the mixture into the prepared pan. Bake until dry and
   firm, 40–45 minutes.
6. Let cool completely in the pan on a wire rack before cutting
   into 16 bars.

Maple-Orange Grain-Free Granola

Serves 4

60 ml fresh orange juice
2 tablespoons pure maple syrup
1 tablespoon coconut oil
½ teaspoon ground cinnamon
¼ teaspoon fine sea salt
50 g coarsely chopped raw almonds
65 g raw macadamia nuts
65 g shelled raw pistachio nuts
15 g unsweetened coconut chips
2 tablespoons chopped unsulfured dried apricots
2 tablespoons chopped dates
2 tablespoons golden raisins
Nondairy milk of choice

1. Preheat oven to 170°C/150°C fan. In a small saucepan, heat orange juice, maple syrup, coconut oil, cinnamon, and salt until boiling. Remove from heat.
2. In a medium bowl, combine the almonds, macadamia nuts, and pistachios. Pour orange juice mixture over and toss to coat. Spread evenly on a large rimmed baking sheet.
3. Bake for 15 minutes, stirring halfway through the baking time. Add the coconut chips. Stir and spread to an even layer. Bake about 8–10 minutes more or until nuts are toasted and golden brown, stirring once. Add apricots, dates, and raisins and stir to combine. Spread granola onto a large piece of foil or clean rimmed baking sheet to cool completely.
4. Serve with nondairy milk.

To store: Place completely cooled granola in an airtight container and store at room temperature for up to 2 weeks.

Energizing Drinks and Snacks

Green Gut Smoothie

Serves 2

1 Granny Smith apple, halved and cored
4 stalks celery, trimmed and cut into large chunks
1 small cucumber, peeled
100 g chopped kale
½ lemon, peeled
1 (1.5-cm) piece fresh ginger, peeled if desired
1 (1.5-cm) piece fresh turmeric, peeled if desired, or 1 teaspoon
     ground turmeric
5 g fresh coriander or parsley leaves
¼ teaspoon cayenne pepper (optional)
150 ml water
3 ice cubes

1. In a high-powered blender, combine the apple, celery, cucumber, kale, lemon, ginger, turmeric, coriander (or parsley), cayenne (if using), water, and ice cubes. Start on low speed and gradually increase the speed to high and blend until smooth.

Variations on Green Gut Smoothie:

Indian Green Shake: Add 3 cardamom pods, a pinch of saffron threads, 240 ml almond milk, and 65 g of kale to the blender with the other ingredients. Blend until smooth. Top with crushed pistachios and 1 tablespoon hemp seeds.

Chai Shake: Bring 240 ml of water to a boil. Add 1 teaspoon black loose-leaf tea and 1–2 teaspoons chai spice blend. Steep for 5 minutes. Let cool. Add tea, 1 scoop vanilla protein powder, and an additional 5 ice cubes to the blender with the other ingredients. Blend until smooth.

Chocolate Green Shake

Serves 1

½ frozen banana
250 ml nondairy milk of choice
1 teaspoon honey or ½ packet raw stevia (optional)
1 tablespoon unsweetened cocoa powder
1 scoop vanilla protein powder
40 g baby spinach or baby kale
2 tablespoons hemp seeds
4 ice cubes

1. In a high-powered blender, combine all ingredients and blend until smooth.

Watermelon Cooler

Serves 6 (1 cup each)

3 tablespoons coconut palm sugar
150 ml boiling water
1.5 kg chopped seedless watermelon
50 ml fresh lemon or lime juice
2 sprigs fresh mint
Ice
250 ml club soda or sparkling water
Fresh lemon or lime slices

1. To make a simple syrup, in a small bowl, combine the sugar and boiling water and stir until sugar dissolves. Set aside.
2. In a high-powered blender, blend half of the watermelon at a time until smooth, and strain through a fine-mesh sieve into a large pitcher; discard the solids.
3. Stir in the lemon (or lime) juice, simple syrup, and mint. Cover and chill for at least 4 hours or overnight.
4. To serve, stir watermelon mixture to eliminate separation. Divide among 6 ice-filled glasses. Top with club soda and garnish with fresh lemon or lime slices.

"Linner"

"Linners" are lunch or dinner meals that are to be consumed midday between the hours of 12 and 5 p.m. Here's a wide variety of soups, salads, bowls, and pasta dishes that provide you with delicious, nourishing, and filling food choices to help optimize your gut health. Feel free to add your own touch to them!

Healthy Gut Salad with Ginger-Turmeric Dressing

Serves 2

FOR THE DRESSING

- 50 ml fresh lemon juice
- 1 (3-cm) piece of ginger, peeled and coarsely chopped
- 1 small clove garlic
- 2 teaspoons ground turmeric
- 3 tablespoons extra-virgin olive oil
- 2 tablespoons flaxseed oil
- 1 tablespoon apple cider vinegar
- 1 tablespoon raw honey or ½ packet raw stevia or agave
- ¼ teaspoon fine sea salt
- Freshly ground black pepper to taste

FOR THE SALAD

- 150 g baby kale salad greens mix (or toss together 75 g each baby kale and baby spinach)
- 1 small apple, cored and diced
- 120 g raspberries
- 30 g coarsely chopped pecans, toasted
- Coarse sea salt and freshly ground black pepper (optional)

FOR THE DRESSING

1. In a high-powered blender, combine the lemon juice, ginger, garlic, turmeric, olive oil, flaxseed oil, vinegar, honey (or other sweetener), salt, and pepper. Blend until smooth.

2. In a large bowl, drizzle the salad greens with 2 tablespoons of the dressing; toss to coat. Divide between two serving plates. Top with apple, raspberries, and pecans. Drizzle with additional dressing and season to taste with coarse salt and pepper, if desired.

To store: This recipe makes about 120 ml dressing. Store any leftover dressing in a tightly sealed glass jar in the refrigerator for up to 1 week.

POWER PLAYER

Greens like spinach, kale, and rocket are not just tasty — they are dense in phytonutrients, phytochemicals, vitamins and minerals, fiber, and antioxidants; they are anti-inflammatory and protect neurons, improving cognition and mood.

Kale-Chard Salad with Creamy Cashew Dressing

Serves 4 generously

FOR THE DRESSING

35 g raw cashews

1 (400 g) can diced fire-roasted tomatoes

1 clove garlic, peeled

2 tablespoons extra-virgin olive oil

Juice of 1 lime

¼ teaspoon smoked paprika

½ teaspoon ground cumin

¼ teaspoon fine sea salt, plus more to taste

1 tablespoon pure maple syrup, plus more to taste

2 chipotle peppers in adobo sauce

FOR THE SALAD

1 bunch kale, washed, stem and ribs removed, coarsely chopped

1 bunch Swiss chard, stem and ribs removed, coarsely chopped

½ teaspoon fine sea salt

Juice of 1 lime
2 tablespoons avocado oil
8 radishes, halved and thinly sliced
½ red bell pepper, seeded and diced
½ orange bell pepper, seeded and diced
1 avocado, pitted, peeled, and diced
40 g dried cranberries
40 g goji berries
35 g hemp seeds
35 g roasted sunflower seeds

FOR THE DRESSING
1. In a small bowl, cover the cashews with hot water and soak for 30 minutes; drain.
2. In a high-powered blender, combine the cashews, tomatoes, garlic, olive oil, lime juice, paprika, cumin, the ¼ teaspoon salt, maple syrup, and chipotle peppers. Blend on high until smooth. Add more salt and maple syrup, if desired. Set aside.

FOR THE SALAD
3. Wash the kale and Swiss chard and spin dry in a salad spinner. Place in a large mixing bowl and sprinkle with the salt, lime juice, and avocado oil. Use your hands to massage the leaves for 3–5 minutes or until volume of greens reduces by about one-third (this helps tenderize the kale).
4. Divide the greens among four large plates or shallow bowls. Top with radishes, bell peppers, and avocado. Drizzle with desired amount of dressing. Top with cranberries, goji berries, hemp seeds, and sunflower seeds.

To store: Store any remaining dressing in a tightly sealed glass jar in the refrigerator for up to 1 week.

Falafel Salad with Tahini Dressing

Serves 4

FOR THE FALAFEL

    2 (400 g) cans chickpeas, rinsed and drained

    4 cloves garlic, peeled and crushed

    10 g loosely packed fresh parsley leaves

    10 g loosely packed fresh coriander leaves

    1 teaspoon ground cumin

    1 teaspoon ground coriander

    ½ teaspoon fine sea salt

    ¼ teaspoon freshly ground black pepper

    2 tablespoons coconut flour

    250 ml extra-virgin olive oil

FOR THE DRESSING AND SALAD

    4 tablespoons tahini

    75 ml water

    2 teaspoons fresh lemon juice

    1 small clove garlic, minced

    2 teaspoons extra-virgin olive oil

    1 teaspoon finely snipped fresh dill (optional)

    ½ teaspoon fine sea salt

    ¼ teaspoon freshly ground black pepper

    275 g mixed salad greens

    4 radishes, halved and sliced

    Lemon wedges, for serving

FOR THE FALAFEL

1. In a food processor, combine the chickpeas, garlic, parsley, coriander, cumin, coriander, salt, and pepper. Cover and pulse until finely chopped, scraping down the sides of the bowl as necessary. Add the coconut flour and process, scraping down the sides of the bowl as necessary, just until mixture holds together.
2. Shape the mixture into compact patties about 10 cm in diameter. Repeat with remaining mixture, placing patties on a

baking sheet or large plate as you work. Cover and chill for at least 30 minutes or up to overnight.

3. In an extra-large nonstick skillet, heat the olive oil over medium-high heat. Add the chilled patties and cook for 8–10 minutes, turning once, until golden brown and heated through. (Cook in batches, if necessary, keeping the cooked patties warm in a 90°C/70°C fan oven.)

FOR THE DRESSING AND SALAD

4. In a glass jar with a lid, combine the tahini, water, lemon juice, garlic, olive oil, dill (if using), salt, and pepper (or whisk in a bowl). (Add more water, if necessary, to reach desired consistency.)

5. To serve, arrange salad greens and radishes on four plates. Top each with two falafel patties and drizzle with dressing. Serve with lemon wedges.

Creamy Cauliflower Soup with Crispy Garlic

Serves 2

1 tablespoon extra-virgin olive oil, plus more for drizzling
2 cloves garlic, thinly sliced
1 small head cauliflower, cored and coarsely chopped
475 ml vegetable broth
1 tablespoon fresh thyme leaves, plus more for garnish
½ teaspoon fine sea salt
¼ teaspoon coarsely ground black pepper

1. In a medium pot, heat 1 tablespoon olive oil over medium-high heat. When hot, add the garlic. Cook and stir constantly until just golden, 1–2 minutes. (You want the garlic to be crisp — it will crisp up as it cools — but be careful not to overcook it, as it will turn bitter.) Using a slotted spoon, transfer garlic to a paper towel–lined plate to drain.

2. Add the cauliflower and cook, stirring frequently, until edges start to brown, 3–4 minutes. Add the broth, thyme, salt, and pepper to the pot. Bring to a boil. Cover and reduce heat to low and cook until cauliflower is tender, about 10–15 minutes.
3. Transfer to a blender and blend until completely smooth (or use an immersion blender in the pot).
4. To serve, ladle the soup into bowls and drizzle with a little bit of olive oil. Top with the crispy garlic and additional fresh thyme.

Note: Homemade broth is best, but store-bought is okay, too. For a quick homemade vegetable broth, scrub 1 large yellow onion (do not peel), 2 stalks celery, 2 large carrots (do not peel), and cut all of the vegetables into 3-cm chunks. Chop 1 bunch green onions and lightly crush 8 cloves garlic (no need to peel). In a soup pot, cook the onion, celery, carrots, green onions, garlic, 6 sprigs fresh parsley, 6 sprigs fresh thyme, and 2 bay leaves in 1 tablespoon extra-virgin olive oil over high heat for 5–10 minutes, stirring frequently, until vegetables are slightly softened. Add 1 teaspoon salt and 2 litres water. Bring to a boil. Reduce heat and simmer, uncovered, for 30 minutes. Strain, discarding vegetables.

POWER PLAYER

Thyme is antioxidant-rich, antimicrobial, antibacterial, anti-fungicidal; historically it has been used to treat abdominal upset, respiratory issues, and acne. It contains carvacrol, shown to affect neuron activity and increase feelings of well-being.

Cumin-Scented Black-Eyed Pea Soup

Serves 4

> 120 g dried black-eyed peas
> 1 tablespoon ghee
> ½ teaspoon cumin seeds
> 3 cloves garlic, minced
> 1 tablespoon minced ginger
> 1 medium tomato, diced
> ½ teaspoon ground turmeric
> ¼ teaspoon cayenne
> ½ teaspoon ground cumin
> ½ teaspoon ground coriander
> 1 teaspoon fine sea salt
> 750 ml water
> 1 tablespoon tapioca flour + 1 tablespoon water (optional)
> Chopped fresh coriander

1. One hour before you plan to cook, place the dried peas in a bowl and cover with 5 cm of hot water; drain before using.
2. Preheat an electric pressure cooker on the sauté function. When the pot is hot, add the ghee. When the ghee shimmers, add the cumin seeds and let sizzle for 30 seconds. Add the garlic and ginger and cook, stirring constantly, for 30 seconds. Add the tomato and cook for 1 minute or until softened.
3. Add the turmeric, cayenne, cumin, coriander, and salt and mix well. Add the black-eyed peas and water. Stir to combine.
4. Cover and lock the lid. Select "manual" and adjust pressure to high. Cook for 15 minutes. When cooking time is over, release pressure naturally for 10 minutes, then release any remaining pressure.
5. Stir. If you would like a thicker consistency to the soup, select the sauté function. Combine the tapioca flour with the water until smooth and stir into the soup. Let cook and bubble for 1–2 minutes or until slightly thickened.
6. Top servings with chopped fresh coriander.

Note: If you don't have a pressure cooker, you can make this soup on the stovetop. Soak the beans overnight. Drain right before cooking. Heat a large pot over medium-high heat. When pot is hot, add the ghee. When shimmering, add the cumin and let sizzle for 30 seconds. Cook the remaining ingredients according to the method through step 3. Bring to a boil over medium-high heat. Reduce heat and simmer, covered, for 60–90 minutes or until tender. If desired, follow step 5.

Roasted Garden Vegetable Soup

Serves 4

FOR THE SPICE MIXTURE

1 tablespoon onion powder
1 tablespoon garlic powder
1 tablespoon dried basil
1 tablespoon dried parsley
2 teaspoons fine sea salt
1 teaspoon freshly ground black pepper

FOR THE SOUP

3 bell peppers (red, yellow, orange, or a mix), stemmed, seeded, and very coarsely chopped
2 large carrots, peeled and cut into 5-cm pieces (halve the thicker ends)
1 small eggplant, peeled and cut into 5-cm chunks
1 large yellow onion, cut into wedges
2 small zucchini, halved lengthwise and cut into 5-cm chunks
3 medium tomatoes, cored and cut into wedges
1 large head garlic
75 ml extra-virgin olive oil
500 ml vegetable stock or broth, plus more for adjusting consistency
Aleppo pepper or crushed red pepper
Yogurt or nondairy yogurt (optional)
Snipped fresh basil (optional)
Gluten-Free Naan, for serving (optional) (see page 273)

1. Preheat the oven to 200°C/180°C fan. Line two very large rimmed baking sheets with parchment paper.

2. In a small bowl, combine the onion powder, garlic powder, basil, parsley, salt, and pepper. Mix well to combine.

3. In a very large bowl, combine the bell peppers, carrots, eggplant, onion, zucchini, and tomatoes. Remove the loose and papery skins from the head of garlic. Cut about 1.5 cm off the top of the head to expose the cloves. Place on a square of foil. Drizzle with a little bit of the olive oil and rub to coat. Wrap in the foil and set aside.
4. Pour the remaining olive oil over the vegetables and toss to coat. Sprinkle with the spice mixture and toss again. Divide between the prepared pans and spread in as thin a layer as possible.
5. Place the pans in the oven. Place the foil-wrapped garlic on the oven rack. Roast for 40–45 minutes, rotating the pans from top to bottom and stirring halfway through, until vegetables are tender and lightly browned on the edges.
6. Combine about one-quarter of the vegetables and 150 ml of the stock in a high-powered blender. Squeeze the roasted garlic pulp into the blender and discard the skin. Blend until smooth. Transfer to a large soup pot. Repeat three more times with remaining vegetables and stock. Adjust seasonings and add broth to achieve desired consistency. Season with Aleppo (or crushed red) pepper, if desired. Cook until steaming and heated through.
7. Top with yogurt and basil, if using. Serve with Gluten-Free Naan (see page 273), if desired.

Creamy Celery Root and Asparagus Soup

Serves 4

1 pound asparagus, woody ends trimmed
2 tablespoons extra-virgin olive oil, plus more for drizzling
2 large shallots, peeled and sliced
1 teaspoon fine sea salt, divided
1 large Yukon gold potato, peeled and coarsely chopped
1 medium celery root (300 g), trimmed, peeled, and
　　coarsely chopped
1 litre vegetable broth
¼ teaspoon ground white pepper
Microgreens, for garnish (optional)

1. Slice 3 cm off the tips of the asparagus and reserve.
   Cut the remaining trimmed spears into 3-cm pieces and
   set aside.
2. In a large saucepan, heat the 2 tablespoons olive oil over
   medium heat. When hot, add the shallots and ¼ teaspoon of
   the salt. Cook, stirring frequently, until the shallots soften and
   become translucent (do not brown).
3. Add the asparagus spears, potato, celery root, and vegetable
   broth. Cover and bring to a boil. Turn heat down to low and
   simmer, covered, for 15 minutes, stirring occasionally, or until
   vegetables are tender.
4. Meanwhile, in a medium saucepan, bring 500 ml water
   to a boil.
5. Prepare an ice bath of 100 g ice and 250 ml water in a medium
   bowl; set aside.
6. Add the asparagus tips to the boiling water and cook for
   1 minute, or just until crisp-tender. Use a slotted spoon to
   transfer the asparagus tips from the boiling water to the ice
   bath. Set aside until ready to serve.
7. When vegetables are tender, transfer them in batches with the
   broth to a blender. Blend until smooth (or use an immersion
   blender in the pot). Stir in the remaining ¾ teaspoon salt and
   the white pepper.

8. To serve, ladle the soup into bowls and drizzle with a little bit of olive oil. Divide the asparagus tips among the bowls and float them on top of the soup. Garnish with microgreens, if desired.

POWER PLAYER

Asparagus contains glutathione — a detoxifying compound that breaks down carcinogens and free radicals and may slow the aging process. It is antioxidant-rich; folate-rich, enhancing mental cognition; high in the amino acid asparagine — a natural diuretic and detoxifier that rids body of excess salts; anti-inflammatory; nutrient-dense; high in fiber, vitamins, minerals, phytonutrients, and sulfur-containing compounds; it also helps ward off oxidative stress and break down and flush toxins from the body.

Curried Sweet Potato, Carrot, and Leek Soup with Crispy Chickpeas

Serves 3

FOR THE CHICKPEAS

1 (400 g) can chickpeas, rinsed and drained
1 tablespoon extra-virgin olive oil
½ teaspoon fine sea salt
1 teaspoon smoked paprika

FOR THE SOUP

1 tablespoon ghee
1 small leek, halved lengthwise, washed, and sliced (white and light green parts)
1 medium sweet potato, peeled and cut into 3-cm cubes
1 large carrot, peeled and roughly chopped
2 teaspoons curry powder
¼ teaspoon cayenne pepper
½ teaspoon fine sea salt
250 ml water
1 teaspoon vegetable soup base
1 (400 ml) can coconut milk
Fresh basil, snipped

1. Preheat the oven to 180°C/160°C fan. Pour chickpeas out onto a clean kitchen towel or several paper towels and dry completely. In a medium bowl, toss the chickpeas with the olive oil. Sprinkle with the salt and smoked paprika. Toss to combine. Bake, shaking the pan halfway through the baking time, until chickpeas are crunchy, 50–60 minutes. Allow to cool completely (they will become crunchier as they cool).

FOR THE SOUP

2. In a medium saucepan, heat the ghee over medium heat. Add the sliced leek and cook, stirring frequently, until softened, 2–3 minutes. Add the sweet potato and carrot, and continue to cook, stirring frequently, until vegetables start to soften, 4–5 minutes. Add the curry powder, cayenne, salt, water, and vegetable soup base and stir to combine. Cover and bring to a boil over high heat. Reduce heat to low and simmer, stirring occasionally, until vegetables are tender, 20–25 minutes.

3. Add the coconut milk. Using an immersion blender, puree the soup until smooth. Heat over medium-low heat, stirring occasionally, until steaming and heated through. (Or, carefully blend the vegetables and broth in a high-powered blender. Transfer back to the saucepan and whisk in the coconut milk.)

4. Top servings with the roasted chickpeas and basil leaves.

Spring Veggie Toast with Fennel Gremolata

Serves 3 (2 toasts each)

FOR THE VEGETABLES

1 small fennel bulb, trimmed, quartered, cored, and thinly
    sliced, fronds reserved

4 medium radishes, halved and sliced

6 spears asparagus, trimmed and cut on the bias into
    1.5-cm pieces

1 tablespoon extra-virgin olive oil

Fine sea salt and freshly ground black pepper

2 tablespoons sliced almonds

Juice of ½ lemon

FOR THE GREMOLATA

    2 tablespoons finely chopped fennel fronds
    Zest of 1 small lemon
    1 small garlic clove, finely minced

FOR THE TOAST

    6 slices (1.5-cm thick) regular, whole-grain, or gluten-
        free baguette
    Extra-virgin olive oil
    Flaky sea salt (optional)

FOR THE VEGETABLES

1. Preheat oven to 200°C/180°C fan.
2. Combine the fennel, radishes, and asparagus on a small rimmed baking sheet. Drizzle with olive oil, season with salt and pepper to taste, and toss to coat.
3. Roast vegetables for 15 minutes or until edges begin to caramelize, stirring the almonds in the last 5 minutes of roasting time. Squeeze the lemon juice over the vegetables and toss to combine; set aside.

FOR THE GREMOLATA

4. In a small bowl, combine the fennel fronds, lemon zest, and garlic. Stir well to combine.

FOR THE TOAST

5. Brush both sides of the bread slices with olive oil. Arrange on a small rimmed baking sheet and toast in the oven 8–10 minutes, turning halfway through baking time and watching carefully to avoid burning.
6. Divide the vegetable mixture among the toasted bread slices. Top with the gremolata and a pinch of flaky salt, if desired.

Rosemary Focaccia
with Caramelized Red Onions, Olives, and Rocket

Serves 8

FOR THE DOUGH
420 ml water at 45°C

1 tablespoon molasses

1 packet active dry yeast (2¼ teaspoons)

240 g spelt flour or stone-ground whole-wheat flour

400 g unbleached white bread flour or gluten-free flour blend,
plus more for kneading

2 teaspoons fine sea salt

1 tablespoon minced fresh rosemary

100 ml + 1 tablespoon extra-virgin olive oil, plus additional for
greasing bowl and parchment

Flaky or coarse sea salt

FOR THE ONION TOPPING
1 tablespoon extra-virgin olive oil

1 large red onion, halved and very thinly sliced

¼ teaspoon fine sea salt

¼ teaspoon black pepper

1 tablespoon balsamic vinegar

50 g halved kalamata olives

35 g baby rocket

FOR THE DOUGH
1. In a small bowl, combine the water and molasses. Sprinkle the
   yeast over the top and stir to combine. Let stand until foamy,
   about 5 minutes.
2. Meanwhile, in a large bowl, combine the spelt or whole-wheat
   flour and the bread flour. Whisk in the salt and rosemary. Add
   the yeast mixture and the 100 ml olive oil. Use a wooden spoon
   to stir ingredients until blended. Sprinkle some additional
   bread flour on a work surface and turn the dough out onto it.
   Knead, adding a little flour as necessary to keep from sticking,
   until a smooth, slightly sticky dough has formed, about
   5–7 minutes.

3. Generously grease a large bowl with olive oil. Form the dough into a ball and place in the bowl, turning to coat. Cover tightly with plastic wrap and allow to rise in a warm spot until doubled, 1–1½ hours.
4. Punch the dough down and let it rest for 15 minutes. Preheat the oven to 220°C/200°C fan. Line a 28 × 23 × 5-cm rimmed baking pan with parchment paper and oil it generously. Press the dough into all corners of the sheet pan. Cover with a damp towel and let rise until doubled, 45–60 minutes.

FOR THE ONION TOPPING
5. Heat the olive oil in a large pan over medium heat. Add the onion, salt, and pepper. Cook, stirring occasionally, until onions are tender and caramelized, about 15–20 minutes. Add the balsamic vinegar and cook, stirring, for 1 more minute, scraping up any browned bits from the bottom of the pan.

FOR THE FOCACCIA
6. After the dough has risen the second time, use your fingertips to poke holes all of the way through and all over the dough. Brush with the remaining 1 tablespoon olive oil and sprinkle with some flaky sea salt. Scatter the onion topping evenly over the top of the dough. Scatter the olives evenly over the dough.
7. Bake until golden brown, 25–30 minutes, rotating pan once halfway during the baking time.
8. Let the focaccia cool in the pan on a wire rack for 10 minutes. Sprinkle with rocket. Cut into 8 rectangles to serve.

Note: If you prefer to go gluten-free, use 675 g of gluten-free flour in place of the spelt and bread flour.

Healthy Nachos

Serves 2

200 g stone-ground corn tortilla chips
50 g shredded nondairy cheddar cheese
115 g cooked black beans

½ teaspoon natural Mexican seasoning blend, such as
     Trader Joe's
50 g frozen corn kernels, cooked and drained
1 small Roma tomato, seeded and finely chopped
1 green onion, chopped
Guacamole
Fresh salsa
Romaine lettuce, shredded
Probiotic dairy sour cream, plain yogurt, or nondairy
     plain yogurt
Jalapeño, thinly sliced
Fresh coriander, chopped
Lime wedges

1. Preheat the oven to 190°C/170°C fan. Spread the chips on a
   rimmed baking pan. Sprinkle the chips with the cheese. Bake
   until the cheese is melted, 5–7 minutes.
2. In a small microwave-safe bowl, stir together the beans and
   seasoning blend. Heat in the microwave on high for 30 seconds.
3. Divide the tortilla chips between two plates. Top with bean
   mixture, corn, tomato, green onion, guacamole, salsa, lettuce,
   sour cream, jalapeño, and coriander.
4. Serve immediately with lime wedges.

Note: If you can't find a prepared natural Mexican seasoning, you
can make your own. In a small bowl, stir together 2 teaspoons
ground cumin, 4 teaspoons paprika, 1 tablespoon granulated garlic,
1 teaspoon dried oregano, ½ teaspoon ground chipotle or cayenne
pepper, ½ teaspoon ground cinnamon, and ¼ teaspoon ground
saffron. Store in an airtight container at room temperature for up to
6 months. Stir or shake before using.

POWER PLAYER

Corn is another antioxidant and phytonutrient dynamo; it is high
in fiber and promotes intestinal health. It is a potent detoxifier,
especially ridding the body of heavy metals, and is high in
antioxidants; it has been shown to improve sleep quality, reduce
anxiety, and stabilize blood sugar.

Easy Hummus Wraps

Serves 2

½ teaspoon ground turmeric

50 g hummus

2 almond-flour tortillas or coconut wraps, warmed according to
    package directions

2 tablespoons Thai sweet chili sauce

35 g baby spinach

2 dill pickle spears

1. Stir the turmeric into the hummus until well blended. Spread
   2 tablespoons hummus over each wrap. Top each with 1
   tablespoon sweet chili sauce and half the spinach. Add a pickle
   spear to one end. Roll up and serve.

One-Pan Roasted Asparagus and Brussels Sprouts

Serves 3–4

3 tablespoons extra-virgin olive oil

1 garlic clove, minced

200 g brussels sprouts, outer leaves removed, trimmed and
    halved (for large sprouts, cut in quarters)

½ teaspoon fine sea salt

Freshly ground black pepper

1 bunch thin asparagus, ends trimmed, cut on the bias into
    5-cm lengths

½ lemon

1. Preheat the oven to 220°C/200°C fan. Stir together the olive
   oil and garlic in a small bowl. Line a large rimmed baking sheet
   with parchment paper.
2. Place the brussels sprouts in a large bowl. Drizzle with about
   half of the garlic oil and sprinkle with half of the salt. Season
   with black pepper to taste. Toss to coat. Arrange in a single layer
   on one side of the prepared baking pan. Roast until sprouts

are almost tender and just starting to brown around the edges, about 10–12 minutes. Stir.
3. Meanwhile, in the large bowl, toss the asparagus with the remaining garlic oil, salt, and pepper to taste. Arrange in a single layer on the other side of the brussels sprouts.
4. Roast just until asparagus is tender, about 7 minutes.
5. Toss vegetables together on the baking pan. Squeeze lemon juice over the vegetables.

Grilled Balsamic Portobello Mushrooms with Sun-Dried Tomato-Basil "Mayo"

Serves 4

FOR THE MUSHROOMS
    50 ml extra-virgin olive oil
    60 ml balsamic vinegar
    3 tablespoons chopped onion
    4 cloves garlic, minced
    ½ teaspoon fine sea salt
    ½ teaspoon freshly ground black pepper
    ¼ teaspoon crushed red pepper (optional)
    4 portobello mushrooms, stemmed
    Extra-virgin olive oil
    Lettuce, tomato, and caramelized onions (optional)

FOR THE "MAYO"
    2½ tablespoons Vegenaise
    1 tablespoon finely snipped oil-packed sun-dried tomatoes
    1 tablespoon finely snipped fresh basil

FOR THE MUSHROOMS
1. In a small bowl, whisk together the olive oil, vinegar, onion, garlic, salt, black pepper, and crushed red pepper (if using) to make the marinade.
2. Place the mushrooms in a resealable plastic bag. Pour marinade over. Seal and massage to coat. Place on a plate and marinate in the refrigerator for 1 hour, turning bag occasionally.

FOR THE "MAYO"

3. In a small bowl, stir together the Vegenaise, sun-dried tomatoes, and basil. Cover and refrigerate until serving time.
4. Oil and preheat a grill or grill pan to medium-high. When hot, grill mushrooms for 10 minutes, turning once, or until cooked through and lightly charred around the edges.
5. Serve with more Vegenaise, lettuce, tomato, and caramelized onions, if desired.

Note: To make caramelized onions, heat 2 tablespoons extra-virgin olive oil or ghee in a large pan over medium heat. Add 2 sliced yellow onions. Stir to coat. Sprinkle with a little fine sea salt and stir again. Reduce heat to low and cook, stirring every 2–3 minutes. If the onions start to stick to the pan, add a tablespoon or so of water to the pan, stirring to scrape up any brown bits. Continue this process for 30–45 minutes or until desired doneness. Caramelized onions can be made ahead and stored in the refrigerator in a tightly sealed container for up to 5 days. Reheat as needed.

Simple Indian-Spiced Chickpeas

Serves 2

1 tablespoon coconut oil
1 small yellow onion, finely chopped
2 teaspoons minced fresh ginger
1 jalapeño or serrano pepper, seeded and minced
1 teaspoon ground cumin
½ teaspoon turmeric powder
¼ teaspoon cayenne
1 teaspoon garam masala
¼ teaspoon fine sea salt
2 medium tomatoes, finely chopped
1 (400 g) can chickpeas, rinsed and drained
Nondairy or traditional plain Greek yogurt
Chopped fresh coriander

1. In a medium pan, heat the coconut oil over medium heat. Add the onion, ginger, and jalapeño and cook, stirring frequently, until the onion is softened, about 3–4 minutes.
2. Stir in the cumin, turmeric, cayenne, garam masala, salt, tomatoes, and chickpeas. Cover and bring to a low boil. Reduce the heat and cook, covered, stirring frequently, until bubbling and saucy, 5–6 minutes.
3. Serve topped with yogurt and coriander.

POWER PLAYER

Coconut oil contains MCTs — medium-chain triglycerides — thought to increase energy expenditure, thereby burning fat more efficiently. It also contains lauric acid and monolaurin, which kill harmful pathogens — that is, bacteria and viruses. Because of the controversy around coconut oil and its effect on harmful cholesterol, it is something that should be used in moderation.

POWER PLAYER

Chickpeas are one of the oldest foods in the world, found in recipes dating back 7,500 years. Packed full of manganese, fiber, and protein, these little beans are the perfect addition to your diet. The versatile chickpea helps control your weight, satiates your appetite, and gives your digestion some TLC.

Sweet Potato–Crust Veggie Pizza

Serves 4

FOR THE CRUST
  2 teaspoons + 1 tablespoon extra-virgin olive oil
  1 medium sweet potato, peeled and cut into 3-cm cubes
  45 g almond flour
  25 g nondairy Parmesan cheese
  ¼ teaspoon fine sea salt
  ¼ teaspoon garlic powder
  1 egg, beaten (or equivalent gluten-free vegan egg replacer prepared according to package directions)

FOR THE TOPPINGS

- 2 tablespoons extra-virgin olive oil
- ½ small red onion, thinly sliced
- 2 garlic cloves, minced
- 1 small red bell pepper, stemmed, seeded, and thinly sliced
- 3 button mushrooms, sliced
- 1 teaspoon dried Italian seasoning
- 1 teaspoon red chili flakes
- ¼ teaspoon fine sea salt
- Freshly ground black pepper
- 5 tablespoons tomato puree
- 40 g baby spinach
- 100 g shredded nondairy mozzarella
- Chopped fresh basil (optional)

1. Preheat the oven to 200°C/180°C fan. Line a large rimmed baking pan with parchment paper. Brush the paper with the 2 teaspoons olive oil.

FOR THE CRUST

2. Place the sweet potato cubes in a food processor and process until the texture of coarse salt. Transfer to a medium bowl. Add the almond flour, cheese, salt, garlic powder, and egg. Mix well to combine. Transfer to the center of the prepared pan and shape into a 30-cm circle. Gently brush with the remaining tablespoon olive oil. Bake until dry in appearance and browned around the edges.

FOR THE TOPPINGS

3. In a large skillet, heat the olive oil over medium heat. When hot, add the onion, garlic, bell pepper, mushrooms, Italian seasoning, chili flakes, salt, and pepper to taste. Cook and stir until vegetables have softened slightly, 3–4 minutes (they do not have to cook completely).

FOR THE PIZZA

4. When the crust has finished baking, brush the tomato puree over it and add a layer of spinach. Top evenly with the vegetable mixture and mozzarella.

5. Bake until the cheese is melted, 8–10 minutes. Sprinkle with fresh basil, if using.

Garlic is one of the most medicinal foods: it prevents and reduces the severity of colds and flu, lowers LDL cholesterol, and is anti-inflammatory, high in antioxidants, and a powerful detoxifier. It can clear intestines and aid digestion, keeping us clear-minded and grounded.

Black Bean Burgers (with a Probiotic Punch)

Serves 4

3 tablespoons extra-virgin olive oil, coconut oil, or avocado oil
1 small yellow onion, finely diced
2 garlic cloves, minced
½ teaspoon ground cumin
¼ teaspoon ground coriander
¼ teaspoon chili powder
⅛ teaspoon cayenne pepper
¼ teaspoon ground turmeric
20 g lightly packed baby spinach leaves, chopped
1 (400 g) can black beans, rinsed and drained
50 g shredded carrot
35 g quick oats
2 teaspoons coconut aminos
1 egg, beaten (or equivalent gluten-free vegan egg replacer prepared according to package directions)
⅛ teaspoon fine sea salt
Freshly ground black pepper
Bibb or romaine lettuce leaves
Beet sauerkraut or regular sauerkraut
Guacamole or avocado slices
Pico de gallo or salsa

1. Heat a medium pan over medium-high heat. Add 1 tablespoon of the olive oil to the pan. When hot, add the onion. Cook and stir until onion is almost translucent, 3–4 minutes. Add garlic and continue cooking for 1–2 minutes more. Stir in cumin,

coriander, chili powder, cayenne, turmeric, and spinach. Cook and stir for 1 minute or until spinach is wilted.

2. In a large bowl, mash the beans with a potato masher or pastry blender. Stir in the onion mixture, shredded carrot, oats, coconut aminos, egg, salt, and black pepper to taste.

3. Stir until ingredients are well combined. Shape into four patties. (You may find it easier to do this with wet hands to prevent sticking.) Place patties on a rimmed baking sheet and freeze for 30 minutes to set.

4. Heat a large pan over medium-high heat. Add the remaining 2 tablespoons of the olive oil to the pan. When hot, cook the patties until crisp on the exterior and cooked through, 4–5 minutes per side.

5. Serve burgers in lettuce leaves topped with sauerkraut, guacamole or sliced avocado, and pico de gallo.

Note: Coconut aminos are a good substitute for soy sauce in low-inflammation diets. It adds an umami flavor similar to soy sauce. Look for it in the health food section of your supermarket or at Whole Foods or natural health stores.

POWER PLAYER

Beans are high in fiber, which helps reduce inflammation and removes waste from the body, aiding digestion; they are also high in flavonoids, which control fat metabolism and appetite. The starch in beans provides long-lasting energy and balances blood sugar levels.

Eggplant "Parm"

Serves 4

1 medium eggplant, peeled and cut into 1-cm slices
1½ teaspoons fine sea salt
Extra-virgin olive oil cooking spray
2 eggs (or equivalent gluten-free vegan egg replacer prepared according to package directions)
1 tablespoon water

100 g coconut flour
¾ teaspoon black pepper
1½ teaspoons dried oregano
1 (675 g) jar marinara sauce (no sugar added)
10 g nutritional yeast
1 (200 g) package shredded nondairy mozzarella
Chopped fresh basil

1. Arrange the eggplant slices on a large wire rack set on a large rimmed baking pan. Salt both sides of the slices with 1 teaspoon of the salt. Let stand 1 hour. Wipe the baking pan dry of any liquid expressed by the eggplant.
2. Preheat the oven to 200°C/180°C fan. Rinse the eggplant slices with cool water and pat dry with a paper towel. Generously spray the baking pan with olive oil spray.
3. In a shallow dish, whisk the eggs with the water and the remaining ½ teaspoon salt. In a separate shallow dish, whisk together the coconut flour, pepper, and oregano.
4. Dip each slice of eggplant in the egg mixture, then dredge in the flour mixture. Set each slice on the prepared baking sheet as you work. Very generously spray the tops of the eggplant slices with olive oil cooking spray.
5. Bake for 20 minutes, then flip and generously spray with olive oil cooking spray. Bake for another 15 minutes. Reduce oven temperature to 180°C/160°C fan.
6. Spray a 24.5 × 19 × 4 cm) rectangular baking dish with olive oil cooking spray. Spread a thin layer of the marinara sauce over the bottom of the dish. Cover with a single layer of half of the eggplant slices. Sprinkle with about half of the nutritional yeast and about one-third of the shredded cheese. Top with about half of the remaining marinara. Repeat layers with remaining eggplant, remaining nutritional yeast, and another one-third of the shredded cheese. Top with remaining marinara and remaining shredded cheese. Bake until bubbly, about 25–30 minutes.
7. Sprinkle with chopped fresh basil and serve.

POWER PLAYER

Eggplant is high in fiber, potassium, and vitamins B and C. Its deep-purple skin also has nasunin, a powerful antioxidant that protects brain cells from free-radical damage and helps transport nutrients to cells.

Penne "Alfredo" with Roasted Cauliflower

Serves 4

FOR THE CAULIFLOWER AND PASTA

1 medium head cauliflower, cored and broken into florets
2 tablespoons extra-virgin olive oil
Fine sea salt and freshly ground black pepper
320 g gluten-free or whole-grain penne
Chopped fresh parsley, for garnish (optional)
Crushed red pepper, for garnish (optional)

FOR THE SAUCE

1½ tablespoons ghee
3 tablespoons unbleached all-purpose flour or 3 teaspoons arrowroot powder
475 ml unsweetened almond milk or soy milk
½ teaspoon fine sea salt
¼ teaspoon black pepper
1 teaspoon onion powder
½ teaspoon garlic powder
¼ teaspoon crushed red pepper
10 g nutritional yeast
50 g shredded nondairy mozzarella
1 tablespoon chopped fresh parsley

FOR THE CAULIFLOWER AND PASTA

1. Preheat the oven to 200°C/180°C fan. On a large rimmed baking sheet, toss the cauliflower with the olive oil and season with salt and pepper to taste. Roast, stirring once or twice, until florets are tender and lightly browned on the edges, for 25–30 minutes.

2. Meanwhile, cook the pasta according to package directions; drain and set aside.

FOR THE SAUCE
3. Heat the ghee in a medium saucepan over medium heat. Sprinkle with the flour and cook, whisking, until well blended. Slowly add the almond milk, whisking as you pour. Whisk in the salt, black pepper, onion powder, and garlic powder.
4. Bring to a simmer and cook until thickened, 3–4 minutes. Whisk in the crushed red pepper, nutritional yeast, mozzarella, and parsley.
5. Toss the pasta with the sauce. Divide pasta among four shallow bowls. Top with the roasted cauliflower. Garnish with additional chopped fresh parsley and crushed red pepper, if desired.

POWER PLAYER

Cauliflower is anti-inflammatory and antioxidant-rich, and it contains sulforaphane, which has been found to improve blood pressure and kidney function and to support digestion by protecting the stomach lining. It has choline, a B vitamin known to boost cognitive function, learning, and memory; and vitamin C to support the immune system.

Black Bean and Sweet Potato Bowls

Serves 2

FOR THE SWEET POTATOES
1 medium sweet potato, peeled and cut into 1.5-cm cubes
1 tablespoon extra-virgin olive oil
¾ teaspoon cumin seeds
⅛ teaspoon cayenne
¼ teaspoon fine sea salt
Freshly ground black pepper

1 tablespoon extra-virgin olive oil

1 clove garlic, minced

1 (400 g) can black beans, rinsed and drained

½ teaspoon chili powder

¼ teaspoon fine sea salt

FOR SERVING

Guacamole

Fresh salsa or pico de gallo

Chopped fresh coriander

Lime wedges

FOR THE SWEET POTATOES

1. Preheat the oven to 200°C/180°C fan. Line a rimmed baking pan with parchment paper.
2. In a medium bowl, combine the sweet potato, olive oil, cumin seeds, cayenne, salt, and pepper to taste. Toss to combine. Spread the sweet potatoes on the prepared pan.
3. Bake until sweet potatoes are golden brown on the edges, 15–20 minutes, stirring halfway through the baking time.

FOR THE BEANS

4. Meanwhile, heat the olive oil in a medium pot over medium heat. Add the garlic and cook, stirring constantly, until golden, 1 minute. Add the beans, chili powder, and salt. Cook, stirring occasionally, until the beans are heated through.

FOR SERVING

5. Divide the beans between two bowls. Top with the sweet potatoes, guacamole, salsa, and coriander. Serve with lime wedges.

POWER PLAYER

Black pepper is antibacterial and vitamin-rich. It stimulates the taste buds, signaling hydrochloric acid secretion and improving digestion; the outer layer of peppercorn stimulates breakdown of fat cells, improving energy and metabolism.

Spicy Toasted Quinoa Pilaf

Serves 2 as a main dish; 4 as a side dish

170 g quinoa, rinsed and drained
1 tablespoon ghee
½ teaspoon black mustard seeds
1 teaspoon minced fresh ginger
1 jalapeño or serrano pepper, seeded and minced
1 small yellow onion, finely diced
475 ml vegetable broth
1 large carrot, peeled and diced
½ teaspoon fine sea salt
1 teaspoon lemon zest
70 g frozen peas (optional)
Fresh basil for garnish (optional)

1. Heat a large, heavy skillet over medium-low heat. Add the quinoa and spread it around in the pan. Cook, stirring frequently, until all of the water (the residual water left over from rinsing and draining the quinoa) is evaporated and quinoa begins to pop. Continue cooking, stirring frequently, until quinoa is brown and aromatic, about 10–12 minutes total; set aside.
2. In a medium saucepan, heat the ghee over medium-high heat. Add the mustard seeds. Cover and cook, shaking the pan, until you hear the seeds pop, about 2 minutes. Turn the heat down to medium. Add the ginger, jalapeño, and onion and cook, stirring frequently, until the onion begins to turn golden, about 5–6 minutes.
3. Add the toasted quinoa, vegetable broth, carrot, and salt. Stir well to combine. Cover and bring to a boil. Reduce heat to low and cook until liquid is absorbed, about 20 minutes.
4. Stir in the lemon zest and peas, if using. Cover and let stand 5 minutes.
5. Fluff with a fork and serve.
6. Sprinkle with fresh basil, if desired.

Peppers contain capsaicin, which fights inflammation and can rev up metabolism and energy levels, reduces pain associated with inflammation, boosts immunity, and clears congestion.

Roasted Cauliflower Tacos with Spicy Chipotle Sauce

Serves 4

FOR THE CAULIFLOWER

    2 teaspoons ground cumin
    2 teaspoons chili powder (mild, medium, or hot)
    2 teaspoons smoked paprika
    ¾ teaspoon fine sea salt
    1 teaspoon turmeric
    2 medium heads cauliflower, cored and chopped into
        1.5-cm pieces
    50 ml extra-virgin olive oil

FOR THE SAUCE

    4 cloves garlic, unpeeled
    35 g raw almonds
    1 (400 g) can diced fire-roasted tomatoes
    1 clove garlic, peeled
    1 tablespoon extra-virgin olive oil
    Juice of 1 lime
    ¼ teaspoon smoked paprika
    ½ teaspoon cumin
    ¼ teaspoon fine sea salt
    1 tablespoon pure maple syrup
    2 chipotle peppers in adobo sauce

FOR SERVING

    8 almond flour tortillas or cassava flour hard taco shells,
        warmed according to package directions
    Lime wedges

OPTIONAL TOPPINGS
   Chopped fresh coriander, thinly sliced red cabbage,
      roasted pepitas

FOR THE CAULIFLOWER

1. Preheat the oven to 200°C/180°C fan. Line a very large
   rimmed baking pan with parchment paper (or use two pans if
   you don't have a very large pan). In a small bowl, combine the
   cumin, chili powder, smoked paprika, sea salt, and turmeric.
   Stir to mix well.
2. Place the cauliflower in a large bowl and drizzle with the oil.
   Toss to coat. Sprinkle with the spice mixture and toss well to
   coat. Spread cauliflower on the parchment-lined pan. Roast on
   the bottom oven rack for 20–25 minutes, or until tender and
   lightly browned on the edges, stirring once.

FOR THE SAUCE

3. While cauliflower is in the oven, roast the unpeeled garlic
   cloves and almonds on another rimmed baking pan on the
   middle oven rack until both are lightly browned and fragrant,
   about 8–10 minutes (watch that the almonds don't burn — the
   garlic may need an additional 4–5 minutes). Remove from the
   oven and allow to cool slightly.
4. Squeeze the roasted garlic cloves into a blender container.
   Add the toasted almonds, tomatoes, peeled garlic clove, olive
   oil, lime juice, smoked paprika, cumin, salt, maple syrup, and
   chipotle peppers. Blend until smooth, scraping down the sides
   of the blender.
5. To serve, divide the roasted cauliflower among the tortillas.
   Top with desired amount of chipotle sauce, and any optional
   toppings. Serve with lime wedges.

POWER PLAYER

Tomatoes are antioxidant powerhouses that are dense in vitamins,
minerals, and fiber; they reduce inflammation, aid digestion, and
protect eye health.

Butternut Squash with Toasted Coconut and Mustard Seeds

Serves 4

2 tablespoons coconut oil
1 teaspoon mustard seeds
1 tablespoon minced fresh ginger
2 cloves garlic, minced
1 serrano pepper, seeded and minced
1 teaspoon ground turmeric
1 (900 g) butternut squash, peeled, seeded, and cut in
   3-cm pieces
150 ml water
¼ teaspoon fine sea salt
50 g finely shredded unsweetened coconut, toasted
15 g chopped fresh coriander

1. Heat the coconut oil in a large pan over medium-high heat. Add the mustard seeds. Cover and cook, shaking the pan, until you hear the seeds pop, about 1–2 minutes. Add the ginger, garlic, serrano pepper, and turmeric, and cook, stirring, until fragrant, about 1 minute.
2. Add the squash, water, and salt. Reduce heat to medium-low. Cover and cook, stirring occasionally, until squash is almost tender, about 5 minutes. Uncover and cook over medium heat, stirring occasionally, until squash is tender and starting to lightly brown and liquid has mostly evaporated, an additional 5–10 minutes.
3. Gently stir in the toasted coconut. Garnish with coriander.

Veggie Summer Rolls

Serves 4

FOR THE SAUCE
60 g creamy almond butter
1 tablespoon hoisin sauce

1 tablespoon coconut aminos
1 clove garlic, minced
1 teaspoon sriracha
3 tablespoons hot water
¼ teaspoon red chili flakes

FOR THE ROLLS
8 spring roll rice wrappers
1 large carrot, peeled and julienned
1 small cucumber, seeded, peeled, and julienned
½ medium red bell pepper, julienned
40 g shredded purple cabbage
1 medium ripe avocado, peeled, seeded, and thinly sliced
Fresh basil and/or mint leaves
4 butter lettuce leaves, torn in half
Sesame seeds

FOR THE SAUCE
1. In a small bowl, whisk together the almond butter, hoisin sauce, coconut aminos, garlic, sriracha, hot water, and chili flakes. Add a little bit more water, if necessary, to achieve desired consistency. Set aside.

FOR THE ROLLS
2. Fill a large shallow bowl or 23-cm round baking pan with warm water. Place one rice wrapper in the warm water and let stand for 15–20 seconds or until softened. Remove from the water, shake off any excess, and place on a flat work surface. Blot excess moisture with a paper towel.
3. Place a few sticks of carrot, cucumber, red bell pepper, and a sprinkle of cabbage on the bottom third of the rice wrapper. Add a slice or two of avocado, and a leaf or two of basil and/or mint. Lay a lettuce leaf half on the top half of rice roll.
4. Fold in the sides of the roll, then carefully roll up, burrito style, into a very tight roll. Place on a serving plate and repeat with the remaining rice wrappers and vegetables. Cut rolls in half on the diagonal and sprinkle with sesame seeds.
5. Serve with the almond butter sauce.

Avocado is considered a superfood: high in fiber, antioxidants, vitamins, and minerals, especially potassium, which protects the body from cardiovascular disease and stroke and stimulates brain functions like memory and learning; it contains oleic acid, reduces inflammation, and increases nutrient absorption.

Quick Vegan Pho

Serves 2–3

100 g bean thread vermicelli
1 litre no-chicken broth or mushroom broth
1 tablespoon minced fresh ginger
2 teaspoons Red Boat fish sauce
1 tablespoon coconut aminos
¼ teaspoon red pepper flakes
1 stick cinnamon (optional)
1 star anise (optional)
2 large shiitake mushrooms, stemmed and thinly sliced
175 g package firm tofu, cut into 1-cm cubes
1 medium carrot, shredded
25 g sliced green onions
1 head baby bok choy, trimmed and cut crosswise into 1.5-cm-thick slices
¼ teaspoon fine sea salt
Toppings: Fresh bean sprouts; fresh basil, mint, and coriander leaves; and thinly sliced jalapeño pepper
Lime wedges

1. Place the bean thread noodles in a large bowl and cover with hot water. Let soak for 10–15 minutes; drain.
2. Meanwhile, in a large pot, combine the broth, ginger, fish sauce, coconut aminos, and pepper flakes (and cinnamon and star anise, if using). Bring to a boil. Simmer, covered, for 5 minutes. Remove the star anise and cinnamon.
3. Add the mushrooms and tofu. Cover and simmer for 2–3 minutes. Add the carrot, green onions, bok choy, and salt.

Simmer just until the bok choy wilts and the soup is heated through, 1–2 minutes. Stir in the noodles.

4. Serve with desired toppings and lime wedges.

POWER PLAYER

Onions may make you cry, but they are anti-inflammatory and contain chromium, which regulates blood sugar, thereby de-stressing the body; and they have phytochemicals, which improve immunity.

Okra Masala

Serves 2

> 225 g fresh okra, rinsed and completely dried
> 1 jalapeño or serrano pepper, seeded and coarsely chopped
> 1.5-cm piece fresh ginger, peeled and coarsely chopped
> 4 cloves garlic, peeled
> 2 tablespoons coconut oil, extra-virgin olive oil, or avocado oil
> ½ teaspoon cumin seeds
> 1 small onion, finely diced
> ¼ teaspoon fine sea salt, plus more to taste
> ¼ teaspoon ground turmeric
> ½ teaspoon garam masala
> 1 tablespoon shredded unsweetened dried coconut (optional)
> 1 teaspoon ground cumin
> 1 teaspoon ground coriander
> Chopped fresh coriander

1. Trim both ends of the okra pods and cut into 1-cm-thick slices; set aside.
2. In a food processor or high-powered blender, combine the jalapeño, ginger, and garlic. Blend until very finely chopped.
3. In a medium nonstick pan, heat 1 tablespoon of the oil over medium-high heat. Add the okra and cook, stirring and shaking

the pan frequently, until it is crisp-tender and bright green, about 5–6 minutes. Transfer to a plate and set aside.

4. Add the remaining 1 tablespoon oil to the pan. Add the cumin seeds and cook, stirring frequently, until they begin to pop, about 2 minutes. Add the chili-ginger-garlic mixture and cook, stirring constantly, for 1 minute.

5. Add the onion and the ¼ teaspoon salt. Cook, stirring frequently, until the onion is translucent, 5–6 minutes. Add the turmeric and garam masala and stir to combine.

6. Return the okra to the pan and cook and stir until ingredients are combined and heated through, about 1 minute. Add the coconut (if using), cumin, and coriander, and stir to combine. Season with additional salt to taste, if desired.

7. Transfer to a serving bowl or platter and sprinkle with the coriander. Serve hot.

Mixed Dal

Serves 4

FOR THE DAL

    50 g masoor dal (red lentils)
    65 g moong dal (split green lentils)
    65 g chana dal (split brown chickpeas)
    45 g toor dal (split pigeon peas)
    500 ml water
    2 tablespoons ghee or coconut oil
    1 medium onion, chopped
    1 ripe tomato, diced
    1–2 jalapeño peppers, seeded and minced
    ¾ teaspoons ground turmeric
    ½ teaspoon cayenne
    ½ teaspoon garam masala
    1 teaspoon fine sea salt

FOR FINISHING

    1 tablespoon coconut oil or avocado oil

1 teaspoon cumin seed
1 teaspoon mustard seed
2 whole red dried chilies
½ teaspoon minced fresh ginger
1 clove garlic, minced
10 g chopped fresh coriander
2 tablespoons fresh lime juice

FOR THE DAL

1. Place the masoor dal, moong dal, chana dal, and toor dal in a sieve. Rinse under cool running water. Transfer to a large bowl. Cover with cool water by 5 cm. Soak at room temperature for at least 30 minutes or up to 4 hours.
2. Drain the dals and place in an electric pressure cooker. Add the water and cook at high pressure for 10 minutes, allowing the pressure to release naturally at the end of the cooking time.
3. Meanwhile, heat the ghee in a pot over medium-high heat. Add the onion and cook, stirring frequently, until golden brown. Add the tomato, jalapeño, turmeric, cayenne, garam masala, and salt. Cook for 1–2 minutes more, stirring frequently.
4. Add the cooked dal to the pot. Add enough water to the pot to achieve desired consistency (think a thick soup, like chili). Bring to a boil, then turn the heat down and simmer for 10 minutes.

FOR FINISHING

5. Heat the coconut oil in a small saucepan over medium-high heat. Add the cumin and mustard seeds and stir constantly until the seeds start to pop, about 30 seconds. Add the chilies, ginger, and garlic. Cook and stir until the garlic starts to turn golden, 1 minute. Stir into the dal along with the coriander and lime juice.

Note: You can vary the amounts of the different dals, as long as the total amount is roughly the same.

Moong Dal Kebabs

Serves 4

200 g moong dal (split green lentils)
2 tablespoons ghee or coconut oil, plus more as needed
3 tablespoons whole-milk Greek yogurt
½ teaspoon fine sea salt
1–2 jalapeño or serrano peppers, seeded and minced
1 tablespoon minced fresh ginger
2 cloves garlic, minced
½ teaspoon garam masala
¼ teaspoon cayenne
1 tablespoon finely chopped fresh coriander
25 g gluten-free bread crumbs
Mixed greens (optional)
Chutney of choice

1. Place moong dal in a sieve. Rinse under cool running water. Transfer to a medium bowl. Cover with water by 5 cm, cover, and soak overnight; drain.
2. In a large nonstick pan, heat 1 tablespoon of the ghee over medium heat. When hot, add the drained dal and cook, stirring frequently, until tender but still whole, about 5 minutes.
3. Transfer to a food processor and add the yogurt. Process until mixture is a thick paste, scraping down the sides of the bowl as needed. Wipe out the pan with a paper towel.
4. Transfer dal-yogurt mixture to a bowl and add the salt, peppers, ginger, garlic, garam masala, cayenne, coriander, and bread crumbs. Use your hands to thoroughly mix everything together.
5. Tightly squeeze small portions together into a ball, then flatten slightly to make patties that are about 6 cm in diameter. (You should get 12 patties.) Heat the remaining 1 tablespoon ghee in the pan over medium heat. Fry in batches until browned and crisp, about 5–6 minutes per side, adding more ghee as needed.
6. Serve the kebabs over the greens, if desired, with chutney.

Vegetable-Oats Dosa

Serves 4 (2 dosas each)

70 g rolled or instant oats
40 g rice flour
40 g semolina
5 g finely chopped fresh coriander
1 jalapeño pepper, seeded and minced
2 tablespoons minced red onion
½ teaspoon fine sea salt
¼ teaspoon freshly ground black pepper
½ teaspoon cumin seeds
½ teaspoon minced fresh ginger
60 g whole-milk yogurt
300 ml water
50 g shredded zucchini, carrot, and/or spinach
1 tablespoon ghee or coconut oil, plus more if needed
Chutney of choice

1. Place the oats in a high-powered blender and blend until powdered. Transfer to a medium mixing bowl.
2. Add the rice flour and semolina and whisk well to combine. Add the coriander, jalapeño, onion, salt, black pepper, cumin seeds, and ginger. Stir well to combine. Add the yogurt, water, and shredded vegetables, and whisk very well to combine and ensure there are no lumps. (The batter will be quite thin.)
3. Heat the 1 tablespoon ghee in a cast-iron skillet or griddle or other nonstick pan over medium-high heat. When a drop of water sizzles in the pan, pour a large spoonful of the batter into the center of the pan and spread it to a circle about 20 cm in diameter. Cook until golden brown and crisp and the top looks dry, about 2–3 minutes, then turn and cook for 1 minute or until both sides are golden brown and crisp. (As the dosa cooks on the first side, gently move a thin flexible spatula under the edge around the circumference, moving toward the center as it cooks, to help prevent sticking. Also, if the dosa develops tiny holes in it, that's just fine — the finished texture should be lacy.)

Transfer the cooked dosa to a plate. Repeat with the remaining batter, adding more ghee to the pan as needed.

4. Serve immediately with chutney.

Quick and Easy Dhokla (Savory Chickpea-Flour Cakes)

Serves 4

Extra-virgin olive oil spray
100 g chickpea flour
½ teaspoon baking soda
½ teaspoon fine sea salt
1 teaspoon cumin seeds
60 g whole-milk yogurt or nondairy yogurt
175 ml water
Optional toppings: black mustard seeds, sesame seeds, and/or red chili powder

1. Spray four ramekins with olive oil spray; set aside.
2. Place a steamer basket in a large, heavy-bottomed saucepan with a lid. Add water to come just below the bottom of the steamer basket. Cover and place over high heat until boiling.
3. Meanwhile, in a medium bowl, combine chickpea flour, baking soda, salt, and cumin seeds. Whisk to combine. Add the yogurt and water and whisk until completely smooth — be sure there are no lumps. (Be sure the water in the Dutch oven is boiling before you add the liquids to the dry mixture.)
4. Quickly divide the batter among the prepared ramekins. Very carefully place the ramekins in the steamer basket, distributing them evenly for weight and setting them so they are as flat as possible. Cover the pot and turn the heat down to medium. Steam for 10–12 minutes, or until a toothpick inserted into the center comes out clean. (There will be a few moist crumbs on the toothpick, but there should not be any liquid batter.)
5. Using the handle on the steamer basket, very carefully remove the ramekins from the pot. Let cool for 5 minutes in the ramekins. Run a sharp knife around the edge of the cakes and turn out onto a serving plate. Sprinkle with desired toppings and serve.

Deconstructed Samosa

Serves 2 as a main dish; 4 as a side dish

2 tablespoons coconut oil
4 medium red potatoes, peeled and cut in 1.5-cm dice
    (about 350 g)
1 tablespoon ghee
1 teaspoon cumin seeds
1 small yellow onion, diced
1 serrano pepper, seeded and minced
1 tablespoon minced fresh ginger
1 teaspoon ground coriander
1 teaspoon garam masala
½ teaspoon fine sea salt
½ teaspoon freshly ground black pepper
¼ teaspoon cayenne
140 g frozen green peas
Nondairy or traditional plain yogurt (optional)
Fresh coriander, chopped

1. In a medium nonstick pan, heat the coconut oil over medium heat. Add the potatoes and cook, stirring frequently, until tender and lightly browned, about 20 minutes. Remove the potatoes from the pan and set aside.
2. Add the ghee to the pan. When hot, add the cumin seeds and cook, stirring constantly, for 1 minute. Add the onion, serrano, and ginger, and cook, stirring frequently, until the onion has softened, 3–4 minutes. Add the coriander, garam masala, salt, pepper, and cayenne. Cook and stir for 1 minute. Add the peas and cook, stirring occasionally, for 1–2 minutes. Return the potatoes to the pan and cook, stirring frequently, until peas are cooked and bright green and everything is heated through, 4–5 minutes.
3. Drizzle with yogurt, if using. Sprinkle with coriander and serve.

Sides

Cheesy Cauliflower Hash Browns

Serves 4 (2 patties each)

Extra-virgin olive oil
1 (350 g) microwavable package cauliflower crumbles
1 egg, beaten (or equivalent gluten-free vegan egg replacer
   prepared according to package directions)
3 tablespoons finely diced red onion
¼ teaspoon fine sea salt
¼ teaspoon black pepper
50 g shredded nondairy or traditional cheddar or mozzarella
5 g chopped fresh coriander
1 tablespoon nutritional yeast
½ jalapeño pepper, seeded and finely chopped
1 clove garlic, minced
1 tablespoon almond flour
⅛ teaspoon cayenne (optional)
⅛ teaspoon ground turmeric (optional)
Extra-virgin olive oil cooking spray

1. Preheat the oven to 200°C/180°C fan. Line a rimmed baking
   pan with parchment paper. Generously grease the parchment
   with olive oil; set aside.
2. Pierce the bag of cauliflower crumbles in a few places with a
   fork. Microwave on high for 4 minutes. Let stand 1 minute.
   Open the package and turn cauliflower out onto a clean cotton
   kitchen towel; allow to cool.
3. When cool enough to handle, wrap the cauliflower up in the
   towel, then twist and squeeze tightly over the sink to get rid of
   excess liquid.
4. Transfer the cauliflower to a mixing bowl. Add the egg, onion,
   salt, pepper, cheese, coriander, nutritional yeast, jalapeño, garlic,
   almond flour, and cayenne and turmeric (if using). Use your
   hands to mix well until you create a dough-like consistency.

Shape into 8 round patties that are about 7.5 cm in diameter, placing them on the prepared baking sheet and flattening to about 1-cm thick as you go.

5. Spray generously with olive oil spray. Bake for 15 minutes or until lightly browned and crispy. Carefully turn and bake an additional 8–10 minutes or until browned and crispy.

POWER PLAYER

Nutritional yeast is trending these days because it is so high in B-complex vitamins, folate, iron, selenium, zinc, amino acids, and fiber. It helps our immunity, is probiotic, and aids digestion; its cheesy-like taste is a great substitute for the real thing, and it is high in protein: 2 tablespoons have 9 grams of protein!

Gluten-Free Naan

Makes 6–8 naan

250 g all-purpose gluten-free flour blend (be sure the blend
  contains xanthan gum, which helps provide structure)
30 g superfine almond flour
2 teaspoons psyllium husk powder
1 teaspoon baking soda
¾ teaspoon fine sea salt
250 ml water at 45°C
1 teaspoon raw honey
1 packet (2¼ teaspoons) instant yeast
60 g plain whole-milk yogurt or nondairy yogurt
½ teaspoon apple cider vinegar
1 tablespoon ghee, melted, plus additional for brushing
Extra-virgin olive oil cooking spray

1. In the bowl of a stand mixer fitted with the paddle attachment, combine the gluten-free flour, almond flour, psyllium husk powder, baking soda, and salt. Turn on low to mix the ingredients. (You can also use a large mixing bowl and a hand mixer.)
2. In a medium bowl combine the warm water, honey, and yeast. Whisk until combined and let stand until foamy, about 5–6

minutes. Add the yeast mixture, yogurt, vinegar, and the 1 tablespoon ghee to the flour mixture. Turn on low, then increase the speed to medium-high and mix for about 4 minutes or until dough resembles thick cookie dough. Use an oiled spatula to shape the dough into a ball. Cover and let rise for 35–40 minutes.

3. Lay a large piece of waxed paper on a work surface. Spray with extra-virgin olive oil cooking spray. Take about 30 g of the dough and roll it into a ball. Place it on the waxed paper and top with another piece of oiled waxed paper. Roll the dough to a 6-cm thickness.

4. Preheat a heavy-duty nonstick pan (such as cast iron) over medium-high heat for 1–2 minutes. When a drop of water sizzles on the pan, remove the top piece of waxed paper and carefully flip the dough onto your hand. Peel off the bottom sheet and, working quickly, place the dough in the preheated pan. Cook for 3–4 minutes or until golden. Flip and cook for an additional 2–3 minutes. Remove to a plate and brush with melted ghee. Cover lightly with foil to keep warm. Repeat with remaining dough, using fresh waxed paper every time. (Naan can be microwaved for a few sections to warm and make pliable again.)

Punjabi-Style Cabbage

Serves 3

1 (3-cm) piece fresh ginger, peeled and cut into chunks
2 cloves garlic, peeled
1 small jalapeño pepper, stemmed, seeded, and coarsely chopped
1 teaspoon garam masala
½ teaspoon turmeric
⅛–¼ teaspoon cayenne
60 ml water, divided
1 tablespoon coconut oil
1½ teaspoons black mustard seeds
1½ teaspoons coriander seeds
½ teaspoon cumin seeds
1 stick cinnamon
1 small yellow onion, thinly sliced

450 g thinly sliced green cabbage
½ teaspoon fine sea salt
Chopped fresh coriander (optional)

1. In a small food processor or blender, combine the ginger, garlic, jalapeño, garam masala, turmeric, cayenne, and 2 tablespoons of the water. Cover and process until smooth, scraping down the sides of the bowl; set aside.
2. In a large skillet, combine the coconut oil, mustard seeds, coriander seeds, cumin seeds, and cinnamon stick. Cook over medium-high heat, stirring and shaking the pan frequently, for 2–3 minutes or until the cinnamon stick unfurls. (The mustard seeds will pop and spatter as they cook.) Reduce the heat to medium and add the onion; cook and stir for 4–5 minutes or until lightly browned. Add the ginger mixture. Cook for 5–6 minutes more or until mixture is nicely caramelized, stirring often.
3. Add the cabbage, salt, and the remaining 2 tablespoons water; mix well. Cover and cook about 8–10 minutes or until cabbage is crisp-tender, stirring twice and scraping up any browned bits from the bottom of the pan. Uncover and cook, stirring frequently, until cabbage is lightly browned and excess moisture evaporates, 3–4 minutes.
4. Remove the cinnamon stick. Sprinkle with coriander to serve, if desired.

Quick Snacks to Go

APPLE: Sliced apple sprinkled with cinnamon. Eat with 2 tablespoons of almond butter.

PROTEIN BARS: There are so many great options out there; just pick one with low sugar (less than 5 grams). Some of my favorite brands: Quest, Combat Crunch, Hemp Force, Golden Ratio, FitJoy.

AVOCADO TOAST: A tablespoon or two of avocado spread on a piece of sprouted gluten-free bread.

Dessert

Salted Zucchini Brownies

Makes 16 brownies

Extra-virgin olive oil spray

250 g creamy natural almond butter

150 g shredded zucchini (2 small)

1 (150 g) bittersweet chocolate baking bar (60% cacao), melted

1 tablespoon unsweetened cocoa powder

1 tablespoon ground flaxseed

5½ tablespoons raw honey

1 egg, beaten (or equivalent gluten-free vegan egg replacer prepared according to package directions)

1 teaspoon pure vanilla extract

1 teaspoon baking soda

½ teaspoon flaked sea salt, such as Maldon, plus more to taste

1. Preheat the oven to 180°C/160°C fan. Spray an 20 × 20-cm baking pan with olive oil spray.
2. In a large bowl, combine the almond butter, zucchini, melted chocolate, cocoa powder, flaxseed, honey, egg, vanilla, and baking soda. Stir well to thoroughly combine. Pour the batter into the prepared pan and smooth the surface with a spatula. Sprinkle the ½ teaspoon salt over the top of the batter.
3. Bake for 35–40 minutes, or until a toothpick inserted into the center of the pan comes out clean.
4. Sprinkle with additional salt, if desired. Let cool completely in the pan on a wire rack before cutting into 16 brownies.

Simple Dessert Choices

Very simple, easy desserts can reward you for a long day's work without sabotaging your energy. My favorites (pick only one):

- 12–16 frozen dark chocolate chips
- 1 spoonful of almond butter
- 100 g of frozen berries mixed with stevia in the blender for a refreshing sorbet
- 5 almonds and 5 chocolate chips
- A piece of chocolate protein bar like Quest, FitJoy, Combat Crunch, or Golden Ratio bars

Cannoli Parfaits

Serves 4

225 g nondairy ricotta
1 tablespoon honey or 2 packets raw stevia
½ teaspoon pure vanilla extract
⅛ teaspoon ground cinnamon
1 teaspoon lemon zest
1 tablespoon nondairy milk
16 raspberries
40 g semisweet mini chocolate chips
40 g coarsely chopped roasted unsalted pistachios

1. In a medium bowl, combine the ricotta, honey, vanilla, cinnamon, lemon zest, and nondairy milk. Stir well until smooth and creamy.
2. Divide half of the mixture among four small parfait or other glasses. Top each with four raspberries and about 1½ teaspoons each of the chocolate chips and pistachios. Top with remaining ricotta mixture, chocolate chips, and pistachios.

To store: Parfaits may be covered and refrigerated for up to 4 hours before serving.

Chai-Spiced Chocolate Pudding

Serves 2

250 ml full-fat coconut milk
60 g chia seeds
1 tablespoon unsweetened cocoa powder
¾ teaspoon chai spice blend
⅛ teaspoon fine sea salt
2 teaspoons honey or agave or 1 packet raw stevia
¼ teaspoon pure vanilla extract
Optional toppings: Ground cinnamon and fresh raspberries

1. In medium bowl, whisk together coconut milk, chia seeds, cocoa powder, chai spice blend, salt, honey, and vanilla. Divide between two small serving glasses or bowls.
2. Cover and refrigerate at least 2 hours or overnight.
3. Dust with ground cinnamon and top with raspberries, if desired.

Note: If you can't find prepared chai spice blend, you can make your own. In an airtight container or glass jar with a lid, combine 3 tablespoons ground cinnamon, 1 tablespoon ground cardamom, 1 tablespoon ground ginger, 1½ teaspoons ground allspice, 1½ teaspoons ground cloves, and 1½ teaspoons ground nutmeg. If you like a little heat, add a few grinds of black pepper. Store at room temperature.

10

Ener-chi

WHEN I WAS GROWING UP with Ayurveda (which means the "science of life" in Sanskrit) all around me, I totally shunned it. I wouldn't be caught dead gargling with a mixture of turmeric, salt, and black pepper for a cold, and when my mom made me a mix of ghee, jaggery (raw sugar), and nuts as an "energy tonic" after my first child — I gagged. And really, for a long time, I pushed this holistic view off to the side . . . until I began my journey of searching for better health and energy.

When I first started on my health plan, I was doing intermittent fasting, I was eating all the right foods, and I was exercising optimally. I noticed I was getting really good at this physical part of my wellness: I was strong and fit, and I had really conquered gut health. But one area that seemed lacking was my mental health. I didn't seem to have a handle on my moods and stress levels, which of course depleted my energy.

When I started getting knee-deep in my research about inflammation, my thinking about what seemed like antiquated old wives' tales went out the window. I realized that the ancient Indian holistic medical system (1) was established by highly spiritual and intellectual sages to foster the balance of mind, body, and spirit that promoted overall health and encouraged compassion for one another, and (2) has been backed up with modern science. It was a toolkit that past generations used to live life to the fullest and to our best potential — something we could all use today. And with reading all this research, I realized our energy is not just our mitochondria or our hormones. It's really a cluster of many different factors — both physical and mental — we have yet to understand. Yet there is so much intuitive understanding of this mind-body connection that has been around for thousands of years.

Much of the "cutting-edge" science about inflammation that we are reading today had already been established in the science of Ayurveda 3,000 years ago. In Ayurveda, they believe in balancing all the life forces and that when things are out of balance — *voilà* — symptoms of inflammation like fatigue, bloating, heartburn, joint pain, or anxiety appear. I'm talking about the Eastern philosophy's embrace of the mind-energy connection, one that, although it has gained prominence in the cultural zeitgeist, is still sorely missing in Western medical practice. The belief that our energy is part of a universal energy that flows in and around the body has been a popular concept for thousands of years in Eastern cultures — take the Hindu prana or Chinese chi. Whatever you call it, there is a long-standing belief that this energy can be increased by thinking good thoughts or doing good works — all actions that happen outside the physical constraints of energy in Western thinking — and if we can access this "inner energy," it will help improve our overall energy and well-being.

Today, as a Western-trained physician, I don't claim to be an Ayurvedic sage, but I do like to incorporate a few things that both Ayurveda and modern medicine agree on: taking a 360-degree approach to our health. While the previous chapters have highlighted how we can improve our energy levels through our food and eating patterns, in this chapter I want to share ways we can boost our energy outside of traditional Western thinking. We have to understand how interconnected our lives are with one another — not just with other people, but with the physical world. Our health depends on what's outside our own bodies just as much as what's within — like our environment and the community of people we surround ourselves with.

Following are some ways to bridge that gap, helping us to feel present, reduce stress, and give an overall sense of well-being. Once you start integrating these in your daily life along with the WTF plan, well, you might just be asking yourself, *How the eff did I get so happy?*

If there's one thing I've learned from Ayurveda, it's that the mind-body connection is something you need to work on *every single day.* Good health includes not just the body but the mind and the spirit. Luckily, the scientific research is now providing more and more evidence of the role the mind plays in our health — the science is helping to push what was considered too "woo-woo" into the mainstream.

Without getting too much into the nitty-gritty, we now know from numerous studies that there is a neural connection between the cerebral cortex and the adrenals responsible for the fight-or-flight response to stress. There is a direct mind-body connection that links how stress, depression, and other mental states can translate into physical ailments and conditions.[1] We also know that there is a direct brain-gut connection. Scientists have found what they call the "*second* brain" — the enteric nervous system (ENS), which are two thin layers of more than 100 million nerve cells lining the entire gastrointestinal tract. It is not capable of thought, but it exchanges signals back and forth with our brain. This is why so many people with anxiety and depression also have IBS and other GI issues.[2]

Bottom line: our chemistry and biology impact our moods, thoughts, and emotions, which in turn all play a major role in influencing our stress, energy levels, and overall physical health. Have you ever felt your stomach tighten up when you were anxious, like having to speak in public or have a difficult conversation with a loved one? That is the mind-body connection at work.

We need to connect our minds to our bodies and find a balance, and it has to be a daily practice, or we will lose that balance (and all that needed energy to get us through the day). Even more than that, we need to keep that energy balance to lift us up and give us joy every day for a lifetime.

There are several things that you can do to ensure this balance.

DON'T GIVE AWAY YOUR
ENERGY FOR FREE

It's a twenty-first-century problem: in today's fast-paced environment, we give away our energy WAY. TOO. EASILY. There's the energy we deplete by running to an important meeting or racing through a supermarket to get dinner on the table, or even the obvious energy we use up when we exercise.

But what I'd like to talk about are the daily events that we don't really think about but that quietly drain our energy resources — like fretting over finances, worrying over a test, or taking way too long to decide what to wear in the morning. And now I want you to think of this energy like money in a bank. Every time you use your energy, you are withdrawing from the bank; the more energy you take out without depositing any, the sooner your bank account is depleted. Your body will give you the signal of INSUFFICIENT FUNDS by feeling exhausted. You wouldn't give your money away for nothing, right? We should be charging a premium for every time our energy is required. Anytime you give a thought or person any kind of attention, you give away your energy. And when that person or thought is negative, it's like draining that bank account. You use up your very precious emotional energy, and then that energy isn't there when you really need it.

You are not alone, either: A 2015 study of 18,000 people across 183 countries found that 68 percent of people yearned to get more rest. More than half of physicians suffer from some form of burnout. Everyone is giving away all their energy, and they are feeling the pain. Let's conserve our energy more wisely and use it when it matters.

When I first started seeing energy as something we should cherish and protect, and I realized my own power in controlling those energy reserves, I made a list. Two lists really: what's "in" — things that brought me joy and replenished me; and what's "out" — things I dreaded doing and that depleted my energy. So things that made me feel energized were on my "in" list, which included spending time with friends and family who energize me, being in nature, and doing yoga.

What was out? The first thing on the list was shopping, for one — I hate shopping. I seriously wear the same five outfits to work every week. I can't be bothered. So now, I either outsource shopping to my husband, who actually loves it, or I buy what I need online to minimize my time. Confession: I also don't love cooking. It's not that I don't like making healthy meals for myself and my family, but I don't like toiling away in the kitchen. I used to think that as a woman, I had to be really into cooking, but I realized that I was depleting energy by even fretting about it. Maybe you are like me — that is why the recipes in this book are very easy! Finally, a biggie on the "out" list: toxic people. I used to feel obligated to engage with certain friends, family, and colleagues who were exhausting to be around. Whether they were just negative people or outright horrible human beings — we all have them in our lives — I chose to engage as little as possible with them.

Once I implemented my "in" and "out" lists in my daily life, I immediately saw huge changes. I was less easily rattled by the small infractions of daily life, less snippy, and more relaxed.

≈

Repeat after me: don't give away your energy on the little, meaningless things that don't warrant it. (As the saying goes, "Don't sweat the small stuff.") Take stock where this kind of energy drain goes and make a concerted effort to stop the leakage. Learn to charge a premium for your energy.

I see these energy "withdrawals" as taking four hidden forms:

1. We drain our energy when we engage with negative people.
2. We drain our energy on negative thoughts.

3. We drain our energy when we eat negative foods.
4. We drain our energy when we are constantly making decisions.

Energy Drain: Negative People

Everyone has that one person in their life who just sucks the energy out of the air. Maybe it's an old high school friend or a cranky uncle. Or maybe it's a colleague who just complains all the time; nothing is right in their eyes. They talk about their problems, then dump their issues on you, leaving little time for you to vent or release your own stress. Their negative energy drains everyone else's — leaving those around them tired, stressed, and confused. Take a tally of your social circle and colleagues as well as your family circle — who zaps your energy? Limit engagement with these kinds of people. Okay, that might be easier with a professional colleague, but how about if this Debbie Downer is in your family? I get it — it is hard to avoid a family member, but do try to limit your time with them or change your engagement with them. Offer little in terms of your own energy.

Think about who gives you energy: Your partner? Your kids? Your best friend? Your dog? Surround yourself with those people — and animals — who are true energizers. These are people who give off positive energy. They are good for you, and you are good for them.

Energy Drain: Negative Thoughts

With the rise of social media, we have been bombarded with more and more news — mostly negative — than we ever have been before as a society. And Facebook, Instagram, and Twitter, among other platforms, have made us engage with the world in new ways. Many of these social media platforms, while initially created to foster a sense of community, can foster an environment of negativity, tribalism, and one-upmanship — all of which can create deep-seated insecurities if we are not careful. Keeping engaged in the virtual world can sometimes be more of an energy suck than the real one. You engage with negative people, ideas, and news cycles, and then you use up your precious emotional energy and you feel depleted, right? So do something that best-selling self-help author Tim Ferriss has done: he has taken a social media "fast," which he claims has made him happier and less reactive. He fasts from social media at least once a week, giving himself screen-free Saturdays.[3] I would add to that advice to take a fast from TV: a few times a week, don't mindlessly watch negative things (ahem, cable news) on TV. Get out of that negativity bubble as much as you can — there is a beautiful world out there.

Quick, Daily Tune-ins

Tuning in doesn't require hours of meditation or yoga (although I do love my yoga); it can be done in as little as five minutes a day. You can simply do anchoring breaths twice a day for two minutes. What that means is having a brief break from whatever you are doing to take deep, slow breaths to anchor yourself in what you are feeling at that moment. Feel your body and listen to what it is telling you, instead of ignoring it. Slow down your breath, make it more even. If you can do this twice a day (at least once in nature, ideally), you are well on your way to a better mind-body connection. This means less inflammatory cytokines and more calming chemicals released into your bloodstream!

Energy Drain: Foods

We talked about food energy wasters before, but it's important to bring them up again so we can see how we waste our precious energy and how we can better think about our choices to preserve that energy — to keep the savings in that bank account healthy.

Think about when you get takeout at lunch or eat dinner at a restaurant. Most restaurants cook with omega-6 oils — corn or vegetable oils — and you know by now that they cause inflammation. To clean up this mess and heal the damage you just did to your gut, you are going to have use a lot of your immune energy. The same goes for sugar and toxins, and (I hate to mention it) even coffee can be a drain to your system. When you have coffee, what you don't realize is that you are "borrowing" energy from your bank. You are going to have to pay it back — by crashing in the afternoon, perhaps sneaking in a nap on the conference room sofa.

This is particularly important for those who have to travel for work: I am constantly told by my patients whose jobs require travel that they feel exhausted no matter what. And it's true — traveling can be so tiring on the body. Being trapped in the extremely dry air of plane cabins, lugging suitcases across football-stadium-sized airports, and just acclimating to a new place — travel drains a lot of energy. Tricia, who travels frequently for her consulting job, had trouble staying consistent with her fasting schedule when she was zipping from one international time zone to another.

Add to that the horrible energy-draining foods available in airports (that salt lick of Delta's chicken marsala. No offense, Delta). So I had Tricia fast through her flights, bringing with her fresh snacks like raw nuts for any hunger pangs. When she landed, she could better acclimate to the new time zone.

Energy Drain: Decision Fatigue

Do you feel you do everything right during the day with your choices, but once you get home, all best-laid plans get pushed aside as you empty the fridge of Trader Joe's bon-bons and slovenly sit on the couch as you rewatch *Friends*? This is what I call going on autopilot when we are tired. We fall back on our innate default pattern of thinking: we reach for what is comfortable when we are tired — that is, comfort food.

There is mental fatigue in every aspect of our lives. A 2011 study that examined judicial rulings by Israeli judges who presided over parole hearings in criminal cases found that judges gave more lenient decisions at the start of the day and immediately after a scheduled break in court proceedings such as lunch. The study showed that the likelihood of a favorable parole ruling peaked at "the beginning of the day, steadily declining over time from a probability of about 65% to nearly zero, before spiking back up to about 65% after a break for a meal or snack."[4]

Short answer: the judges were plumb tired and their critical thinking was zapped midday and later in the day, when they were more likely to be hungry and fatigued from work.

We are better than that. We have another way of thinking, a more complex, deeply thoughtful decision-making process, but it's limited. If you use up this type of thinking early in the day, you can't really get it back. We make dozens of decisions every day. Actually more than that — a study by Cornell University shows that we make 226 decisions a day just on food; other studies indicate that we make about 35,000 conscious decisions *daily*.[5] Considering we sleep for a third of that day, you are looking at about 2,000 decisions an hour. That is crazy!

These decisions range from mundane things like what to wear to serious, thoughtful work decisions. You want to reserve your energy for complex thinking for meaningful decisions. Save your energy for writing that presentation, not worrying about what you are going to wear or what people will think of it. Maximize your energy for big decisions that will move your life forward, and save those decisions for the morning, when your energy banks have been refilled and you can think the most critically.

MAKE DEPOSITS IN THE ENERGY BANK

You can optimize your energy by minimizing and automating where you can — negative thoughts and what you are going to have for breakfast — and maximizing on the bigger, more important tasks at hand. We have talked about how when you eat is important, but timing is also important in your decision-making process.

Energy Optimizers

1. Engage more and plan more things with people who give you energy.
2. Give yourself an energizing hour every day: it could be working out, reading, cooking, anything that recharges your batteries. This is a must!
3. Make a list: five things/people that drain you and five things/people that energize you. Then work on controlling the output of your energy. Don't engage with a person who is draining. Holiday time is an especially hard time for this — protect yourself and don't engage, or at least minimize that time.

All the Right Foods and All the Right Exercise

It bears repeating that eating the right foods, as laid out in this book, will give you great energy reserves. Timing it with exercise and the right sleep patterns will make this a sound investment.

Many of you yogis out there may not need me to tell you how there is a strong mind-body connection with yoga and meditation, and how integrating those practices into your daily life can be life-changing. Studies show that movement and breathing done in yoga wakes up the relaxation response in our vagus nerve and activates GABA, a neurotransmitter in the brain that helps us relax and de-stress. A 12-week study monitored people who walked or did yoga for an hour three times a week. At the end of the study, the yoga group had better GABA levels, along with greater improvement in mood and reduced anxiety.[6] Your body will feel better, your mind clearer, more focused. Trust me.

Guided Imagery and Mindfulness Exercises

There's a lot of evidence that mental imagery can change health outcomes like weight loss and can increase energy. A recent study on people trying to lose weight found that when they used guided imagery, they lost an average of five times more weight than those using talking therapy alone. Visualizing how it will feel, sound, smell, and look like to have lost weight helped them shed pounds.[7] This is a great technique to use to bring yourself down a notch when you need to de-stress and regain energy — there are tons (*tons*) of sites online that provide scripts and videos that can guide you.

And while you are online, check out websites and podcasts about mindfulness. This practice of bringing a nonjudgmental awareness to the present moment can also help enormously in lowering stress levels and refilling those energy stores.

Saunas

I briefly mentioned the sweet spot of saunas in chapter 8, but I include it here, too, as they are a great way to add to your energy bank. Saunas and communal baths have been around for thousands of years as a purification and healing practice in a multitude of cultures. This exposure brings on mild hyperthermia — an increase in the body's core temperature — that in turn "induces a thermoregulatory response involving neuroendocrine, cardiovascular, and cytoprotective mechanisms that work together to restore homeostasis and condition the body for future heat stressors."[8] Translation? It is really good for you! If you can't sit still in a sauna, think about trying hot yoga (one of my favorite ways to enjoy heat-related benefits) or some other movement-based form of heating your core temperature.

In the last several years, sauna use has reemerged as a hot topic (pun intended). Studies have shown that short spurts of heat improve overall health. One study in particular following more than 2,300 middle-aged men from eastern Finland identified strong links between sauna use and reduced death and disease.[9]

Another study showed that sauna use in combination with aerobic exercise can offer additional health benefits. While a high level of aerobic fitness or "frequent sauna use is independently associated with lower cardiovascular-related mortality," this study found that aerobic exercise in combination with frequent sauna bathing is *even better*.[10]

Take a gander at these stats: Several studies have shown that frequent sauna bathing provides a 50 percent lower risk for fatal heart disease, 51 percent lower risk for stroke, and 46 percent lower risk for hypertension.[11] Just a single sauna session has been shown to lower blood pressure, improve heart rate variability, and improve the flexibility of our arteries.[12] Still not convinced? Frequent sauna use is associated with a 40 percent lower mortality and a 60 percent lower risk for Alzheimer's disease.[13]

Nature

The art of Ayurveda is about living in complete harmony with nature as well as with ourselves. I recommend getting a quick dose of nature every day—whether it's a few minutes of sunlight in the morning or taking a quick walk or rolling down the car window on your commute. In a 1989 study from the University of Illinois, researchers found that simply stepping into nature can restore your physical and mental energy. Don't forget that exposure to nature raises our levels of serotonin and melatonin, and increases productivity.[14]

CREATE A SAFE SPACE

Think about it—your home is your castle where you go to relax, right? To kick off your uncomfortable shoes and change into your comfy clothes. You get to wash away the day and spend time with loved ones. And with stress levels as high as they are today, having this sanctuary is more important than ever. However, there are simple and surprising things around you that might make your sanctuary a little less soothing. Here are some tips on how to bring in good energy to your home:

- *Light:* We have talked about artificial lighting and blue light — have you thought about the light that streams in from a streetlamp or your neighbor's house? Or the bright (and obnoxious at three in the morning) numbers on your alarm clock? Think about the lighting that surrounds you and try to bring in as much natural light as possible during the day. At night, use blackout curtains or blinds to get your much-needed sleep.

- *Choose soothing scents, sounds, and decor:* Like lavender? Studies show that it calms, and soft sounds can be soothing, too. I know some people swear by having music playing in the background — jazz, classical, soft electronica, take your pick — to help them focus. Buying new furniture? Choose calm, soothing colors and stay away from sharp angles — studies have shown these angles activate a part of the brain associated with unconscious fear.[15] This may be our brain telling us to watch out, danger ahead (much like it would if it saw a sharp knife or a rough terrain).[16] Further accessorize with lots of green plants. Yes, my WTF plan is centered on a plant-based diet, but I am also big on real plants that reduce anxiety and freshen the air.

- *Declutter:* Love her or hate her, Marie Kondo is right about decluttering your home. I know we are all busy — who has time to tackle that closet? Recent studies show a link between a cluttered home and stress and anxiety.[17] So keep your space clean and tidy as much as you can. As Admiral William H. McRaven said in his best-selling book, "Make your bed." Every day.[18] So simple, but you will feel organized, productive, and ready to tackle the day.

❧

Ayurvedic author Shubhra Krishan succinctly explains, "The Ayurvedic route to great health involves two simple steps: 1. Doing less; 2. Being more."[19] Let that be the takeaway of this chapter — heck, the takeaway of this entire book: let's do everything possible to increase our spiritual, mental, and physical aspects of health. Don't waste your energy on meaningless or trivial things — save it for those times that mean something to you and those people you cherish. With these actionable steps, I hope you'll notice life-changing results in your energy levels and, more important, gain a presence of mind and boost your happiness.

Acknowledgments

This book was just a dream I had when I first started this journey into wellness. A dream I thought I would fulfill someday long after I retired from clinical medicine.

There are too many people to thank here who have supported me, encouraged me, educated me, and inspired me to make that dream a reality.

❧

First off, I have to thank my darling husband, Akshay, who is literally the best thing that has ever happened to me. He allowed me to pursue my dreams while always challenging me on my big ideas. He is the practicality to my passion. In a world where women are asked to be *everything*, he has lifted part of that burden so that I can be my *own thing*. Without him there would be no book. He is a gem. Akshay, I thank you for being my partner on this crazy road called life. I love you and owe this book to you.

To my children, Jaden and Lara, everyone says you are Mini-Mes of your dad and me. But I think you are so much more. You are our best teachers. You hold my heart like no other. I would do anything for you. Seeing you grow up as confident, fun, *happy* people is my life's goal.

To my parents, without your sacrifice of coming to this country, I can confidently say I would not be where I am today. A little girl born in Baroda writing a book is a dream.

To my agent, Heather, thank you for believing in me. Thank you for introducing me to so many amazing people and for being such a great support system throughout this crazy journey. To my collaborator, Kathy, thank you for our deep chats and for help in pulling out what's important to women. I enjoyed learning the nuances of writing and am sorry for all the typos!

❧

To my recipe development team, thank you for taking my ideas and my many restrictions and turning them into reality.

To my editor, Sarah, thank you for our amazing conversations in the early days with Heather. Thank you for being so patient and helpful. I'm so grateful to have met you. To my marketing and publicity team from HMH, thank you for keeping after me when I forget to answer your emails, and thank you for your savviness in getting this book out into the world!

❧

To my brother, Ashil, my sister-in-law, and Kayan — thank you for teaching me what it feels like to be a mom before I actually became a mom! I adore you guys.

To my mother-in-law, father-in-law, sister-in-law, brother-in-law, Sani, and Arjun, I appreciate you opening my eyes to the wonders of California, the beauty of a long sit-down dinner with your family, and your support through all these years.

To my BC friends, thank you for making me laugh and having a sisterhood.

To my Cornell, Binghamton, Einstein, Columbia, Beth Israel colleagues and friends, I think of you often and I'm blessed that so many of us are still in touch. To my Arizona friends and colleagues at Vallen ENT, I have grown so much since moving to Arizona in 2010. I have honestly picked and chosen each one of you, as I learned that positivity is the most important aspect of a friendship. Thank you for being there for me and supporting me through everything. To my gyms, Modern Yoga and BODI Scottsdale, and my trainers, thank you for keeping me sane during this time.

To my family in India, I cherish all those summers that I came to India and was able to spend time with you and learn about our amazing culture.

To the G-team, you guys, especially Latim, are the reason I am here today. I treasure our family and your support. Mital, I can say you are one of the reasons I have broken out of my shell. Thanks for being my sounding board, supporter, and the best sister all around.

To Covid, thank you for teaching us all, especially medical professionals, that we don't know everything, and that we have to have a little patience — and build up our resiliency.

Appendix

A few tests for hormonal imbalance:

- Complete blood cell count: includes white blood cells
- Hemoglobin: looks at blood levels
- Hematocrit: looks at platelet count
- Complete thyroid panel: looks at function of your thyroid, including thyroid-stimulating hormone, which is TSH, a free T4
- Complete lipid panel: includes total cholesterol, triglycerides, LDL, HDL, VLDL, LDL particle size, apo A, apo B, apo A to apo B ratio
- Adrenal panel: measures cortisol levels, DHEA, and DHEA-S
- Complete metabolic panel
- Comprehensive liver function testing
- Glucose and insulin levels
- Hs-CRP test measures the levels of the body's C-reactive protein, which is a good marker for inflammation
- Kidney function tests: includes BUN and creatinine
- Vitamin D_3 levels
- Zinc and ferritin levels
- Calcium levels
- If you're overweight, consider measuring leptin and IGF-1

Notes

INTRODUCTION

1. Scott Hensley, "Annals of the Obvious: Women Way More Tired than Men," NPR, April 12, 2013, www.npr.org/sections/health-shots/2013/04/11/176936210/annals -of-the-obvious-women-way-more-tired-than-men.
2. "QuickStats: Percentage of Adults Who Often Felt Very Tired or Exhausted in the Past 3 Months, by Sex and Age Group — National Health Interview Survey, United States, 2010–2011," *Morbidity and Mortality Weekly Report* 62, no. 14 (April 12, 2013): 275, Centers for Disease Control and Prevention, www.cdc.gov/mmwr/preview/ mmwrhtml/mm6214a5.htm.
3. Yasmin Anwar, "Why Middle-Class Black Women Dread the Doctor's Office," *Berkeley News*, January 18, 2019, news.berkeley.edu/2019/01/18/invisiblevisits/.
4. Rob Haskell, "Serena Williams on Motherhood, Marriage, and Making Her Comeback," *Vogue*, February 2018, www.vogue.com/article/serena-williams-vogue-cover -interview-february-2018.
5. Anwar, "Why Middle-Class Black Women Dread the Doctor's Office."
6. "Gut Microbes from Healthy Infants Block Milk Allergy Development in Mice," National Institutes of Health, US Department of Health and Human Services, January 14, 2019, https://www.nih.gov/news-events/news-releases/gut-microbes-healthy -infants-block-milk-allergy-development-mice.
7. Hans P. A. Van Dongen, Greg Maislin, Janet M. Mullington, and David F. Dinges, "The Cumulative Cost of Additional Wakefulness: Dose-Response Effects on Neurobehavioral Functions and Sleep Physiology from Chronic Sleep Restriction and Total Sleep Deprivation," *Sleep* 26, no. 2 (March 15, 2003): 117–26, available at US National Library of Medicine, https://www.ncbi.nlm.nih.gov/pubmed/12683469.
8. Lawrence A. David et al., "Diet Rapidly and Reproducibly Alters the Human Gut Microbiome," *Nature* 505, no. 7484 (January 23, 2014): 559–63, available at US National Library of Medicine, https://www.ncbi.nlm.nih.gov/pmc/articles/PMC3957428/.

1. WHAT *ARE* HORMONES, ANYWAY?

1. Katherine Wu, "Love, Actually: The Science Behind Lust, Attraction, and Companionship," *Science in the News*, February 14, 2019, Harvard University, http://sitn.hms .harvard.edu/flash/2017/love-actually-science-behind-lust-attraction-companion ship/.
2. "Hypothalamic Dysfunction," A.D.A.M. Multimedia Encyclopedia, Penn State Her-

shey, Milton S. Hershey Medical Center, http://pennstatehershey.adam.com/content.aspx?productid=117&pid=1&gid=001202.

3. Thushani Siriwardhane et al., "Significance of Anti-TPO as an Early Predictive Marker in Thyroid Disease," *Autoimmune Diseases*, July 28, 2019, available at Hindawi, https://www.hindawi.com/journals/ad/2019/1684074/.

4. Geanina Popoveniuc and Jacqueline Jonklaas, "Thyroid Nodules," *Medical Clinics of North America* 96, no. 2 (March 2012): 329–49, available at US National Library of Medicine, https://www.ncbi.nlm.nih.gov/pmc/articles/PMC3575959/.

5. Syed Khalid Imam and Shamim I. Ahmad, *Thyroid Disorders: Basic Science and Clinical Practice* (Cham, Switzerland: Springer International, 2016).

6. "Hyperthyroidism (Overactive Thyroid)," National Institute of Diabetes and Digestive and Kidney Diseases, US Department of Health and Human Services, https://www.niddk.nih.gov/health-information/endocrine-diseases/hyperthyroidism#whoLikely.

7. Lei Zhou, Xinli Li, Ayaz Ahmed, Dachang Wu, Liang Liu, Juanjuan Qiu, Yao Yan, Meilan Jin, and Yi Xin, "Gut Microbe Analysis Between Hyperthyroid and Healthy Individuals," *Current Microbiology* 69, no. 5 (November 2014): 675–80, available at US National Library of Medicine, https://www.ncbi.nlm.nih.gov/pubmed/24969306.

8. "Type 2 Diabetes," diaTribe, https://diatribe.org/type-2-diabetes.

9. "Polycystic Ovary Syndrome (PCOS)," Mayo Clinic, https://www.mayoclinic.org/diseases-conditions/pcos/symptoms-causes/syc-20353439.

10. Karen Weintraub, "'Stress Hormone' Cortisol Linked to Early Toll on Thinking Ability," *Scientific American*, October 25, 2018, https://www.scientificamerican.com/article/ldquo-stress-hormone-rdquo-cortisol-linked-to-early-toll-on-thinking-ability/.

11. Karolina Zaremba, "The Pregnenolone Steal: What Does It Mean for Your Health?," *Fullscript* (blog), https://fullscript.com/blog/pregnenolone-steal.

12. Sara Gottfried, *The Hormone Cure: Reclaim Balance, Sleep, and Sex Drive; Lose Weight; Feel Focused, Vital, and Energized Naturally with the Gottfried Protocol* (New York: Scribner, 2014).

13. Jo Jones, William Mosher, and Kimberly Daniels, "Current Contraceptive Use in the United States, 2006–2010, and Changes in Patterns of Use Since 1995," in *Sexual Statistics: Select Reports from the National Center for Health Statistics* (Hauppauge, NY: Nova Science, 2013), 127–73.

14. Yasmine Belkaid and Timothy Hand, "Role of the Microbiota in Immunity and Inflammation," *Cell* 157, no. 1 (March 27, 2014): 121–41, available at US National Library of Medicine, https://www.ncbi.nlm.nih.gov/pmc/articles/PMC4056765/.

15. University of Illinois at Urbana-Champaign, "Long-Term Estrogen Therapy Changes Microbial Activity in the Gut," *ScienceDaily*, June 19, 2018, www.sciencedaily.com/releases/2018/06/180619173557.htm.

2. HOW DID OUR HORMONES GET SO EFFED UP?

1. Jane E. Brody, "Are G.M.O. Foods Safe?" *New York Times*, April 23, 2018, https://www.nytimes.com/2018/04/23/well/eat/are-gmo-foods-safe.html.

2. Liz Moody, "These 8 Foods Are Wreaking Havoc on Your Hormones," Mindbodygreen, October 7, 2019, https://www.mindbodygreen.com/0-29200/these-8-foods-are-wreaking-havoc-on-your-hormones.html.

3. "Toxic Substances Portal — Polychlorinated Biphenyls (PCBs)," Centers for Disease

Control and Prevention, July 2014, https://www.atsdr.cdc.gov/toxfaqs/tf.asp?id=140&tid=26.

4. J. D. Heyes, "Monsanto Roundup Harms Human Endocrine System at Levels Allowed in Drinking Water, Study Shows," Global Research, April 6, 2015, https://www.globalresearch.ca/monsanto-roundup-harms-human-endocrine-system-at-levels-allowed-in-drinking-water-study-shows/5441051.

5. Chun Z. Yang, Stuart I. Yaniger, V. Craig Jordan, Daniel J. Klein, and George D. Bittner, "Most Plastic Products Release Estrogenic Chemicals: A Potential Health Problem That Can Be Solved," Environmental Health Perspectives 119, no. 7 (July 1, 2011): 989–96, available at US National Library of Medicine, https://www.ncbi.nlm.nih.gov/pmc/articles/PMC3222987/.

6. Chris Kresser, "How Plastic Food Containers Can Make You Sick," ChrisKresser.com, October 27, 2011, https://chriskresser.com/how-plastic-food-containers-could-be-making-you-fat-infertile-and-sick/.

7. UHN Staff, "5 Possible Sources of BPA Exposure," University Health News, April 14, 2020, https://universityhealthnews.com/daily/nutrition/5-alarming-sources-of-bpa-exposure/.

8. Center for Food Safety and Applied Nutrition, "Parabens in Cosmetics," US Food and Drug Administration, FDA, https://www.fda.gov/cosmetics/cosmetic-ingredients/parabens-cosmetics.

9. "4 Harmful Endocrine-Disruptors to Avoid in Beauty Products," Simply Organic Beauty, October 26, 2017, https://www.simplyorganicbeauty.com/avoid-endocrine-disruptors-cosmetics/.

3. ADRENAL FATIGUE IS NOT JUST ABOUT THE ADRENALS

1. Flavio A. Cadegiani and Claudio E. Kater, "Adrenal Fatigue Does Not Exist: A Systematic Review," BMC Endocrine Disorders 16, no. 1 (2016): 48, available at US National Library of Medicine, https://www.ncbi.nlm.nih.gov/pmc/articles/PMC4997656/.

2. "Adrenal Fatigue," Endocrine Society, https://www.hormone.org/diseases-and-conditions/adrenal-fatigue.

3. Zack Guzman, "This Chart Shows How Far Behind America Is in Paid Time Off Compared to the Rest of the World," CNBC, August 15, 2018, https://www.cnbc.com/2018/08/15/statista-how-far-behind-us-is-in-paid-time-off-compared-to-the-world.html.

4. Scott Gavura, "Adrenal Fatigue: A Fake Disease (Updated)," Science-Based Medicine, https://sciencebasedmedicine.org/adrenal-fatigue-a-fake-disease/.

4. INFLAMMATION IS AN ENERGY LEECH

1. Roma Pahwa, Amandeep Goyal, Pankaj Bansal, and Ishwarlal Jialal, "Chronic Inflammation," StatPearls, updated March 2, 2020, available at US National Library of Medicine, https://www.ncbi.nlm.nih.gov/books/NBK493173/.

2. G. E. Dinse, C. G. Parks, C. R. Weinberg, C. A. Co, J. Wilkerson, D. C. Zeldin, E. K. L. Chan, and F. W. Miller, "Increasing Prevalence of Antinuclear Antibodies in the United States," Arthritis & Rheumatology 72, no. 6 (June 2020): 1026–35, available at US National Library of Medicine, pubmed.ncbi.nlm.nih.gov/32266792/.

3. "Asthma in the US," Centers for Disease Control and Prevention, May 3, 2011, https://www.cdc.gov/vitalsigns/asthma/index.html.

4. Society for Neuroscience, "How Inflammatory Disease Causes Fatigue," ScienceDaily, February 28, 2009, www.sciencedaily.com/releases/2009/02/090217173034.htm.

5. Nicola R. Sproston and Jason J. Ashworth, "Role of C-Reactive Protein at Sites of Inflammation and Infection," *Frontiers in Immunology* 9 (April 13, 2018), available at US National Library of Medicine, https://www.ncbi.nlm.nih.gov/pmc/articles/PMC5908901/.

6. Barbara J. Nicklas et al., "Diet-Induced Weight Loss, Exercise, and Chronic Inflammation in Older, Obese Adults: A Randomized Controlled Clinical Trial," *American Journal of Clinical Nutrition* 79 (April 2004): 4, available at Oxford Academic, academic.oup.com/ajcn/article/79/4/544/4690130.

7. Vincent M. Pedre, "5 Signs Your Inflammation Isn't as Under Control as You Think," Mindbodygreen, October 2, 2018, https://www.mindbodygreen.com/articles/5-signs-your-inflammation-isn-t-as-under-control-as-you-think.

8. M. C. Arrieta, L. Bistritz, and J. B. Meddings, "Alterations in Intestinal Permeability," *Gut* 55, no. 10 (October 2006): 1512–20, available at US National Library of Medicine, https://www.ncbi.nlm.nih.gov/pmc/articles/PMC1856434/.

9. Sarah Ellis, "7 Signs You Have a Leaky Gut," Mindbodygreen, updated January 24, 2019, https://www.mindbodygreen.com/0-10908/9-signs-you-have-a-leaky-gut.html.

10. Ramón Estruch et al., "Primary Prevention of Cardiovascular Disease with a Mediterranean Diet," *New England Journal of Medicine* 368 (April 4, 2013): 1279–90, www.nejm.org/doi/full/10.1056/nejmoa1200303.

11. Jennifer Johnson, "Poor Sleep Quality Increases Inflammation, Community Study Finds," Woodruff Health Sciences Center, Emory University, November 15, 2010, http://shared.web.emory.edu/whsc/news/releases/2010/11/poor-sleep-quality-increases-inflammation-study-finds.html.

12. "Study: Stress May Cause Excess Abdominal Fat in Otherwise Slender Women," YaleNews, September 22, 2000, https://news.yale.edu/2000/09/22/study-stress-may-cause-excess-abdominal-fat-otherwise-slender-women.

5. GUT REACTION

1. Brie Wieselman, "Why Your Gut Health and Microbiome Make-or-Break Your Hormone Balance," Brie Wieselman, September 28, 2018, https://briewieselman.com/why-your-gut-health-and-microbiome-make-or-break-your-hormone-balance/.

2. Rhonda Patrick, "How the Gut Microbiota Affects Our Health with Dr. Erica and Dr. Justin Sonnenburg," *FoundMyFitness* podcast, January 3, 2016, https://www.foundmyfitness.com/episodes/the-sonnenburgs.

3. Patrick, "How the Gut Microbiota Affects Our Health."

4. Jennifer Yttri, "Bacteria: The Good, the Bad, and the Ugly," National Center for Health Research, http://www.center4research.org/bacteria-good-bad-ugly/.

5. Emily R. Davenport, Jon G. Sanders, Se Jin Song, Katherine R. Amato, Andrew G. Clark, and Rob Knight, "The Human Microbiome in Evolution," *BMC Biology* 15 (December 27, 2017): 127, available at US National Library of Medicine, https://www.ncbi.nlm.nih.gov/pmc/articles/PMC5744394/.

6. Università di Trento, "Lifestyle Is a Threat to Gut Bacteria: Ötzi Proves It, Study Shows," ScienceDaily, October 18, 2019, https://www.sciencedaily.com/releases/2019/10/191018112136.htm.

7. Erica Sonnenburg, "Microbes Are Holding the Reins to Our Health," *Psychology To-*

day, April 12, 2015, https://www.psychologytoday.com/us/blog/the-good-gut/201504/microbes-are-holding-the-reins-our-health.

8. Sara Gottfried, "Q & A with Chris Kresser," Dr. Sara Gottfried, MD, November 28, 2014, https://www.saragottfriedmd.com/q-a-with-chris-kresser/.

9. "How Your Gut Microbiome Influences Your Hormones," Bulletproof, June 6, 2019, https://www.bulletproof.com/gut-health/gut-microbiome-hormones/#ref-6.

10. Chris Kresser, "The Gut-Hormone Connection: How Gut Microbes Influence Estrogen Levels," Kresser Institute, November 15, 2017, https://kresserinstitute.com/gut-hormone-connection-gut-microbes-influence-estrogen-levels/.

11. Ocean Robbins, "The Surprising Truth About Bone Broth," Food Revolution Network, January 7, 2020, https://foodrevolution.org/blog/bone-broth-benefits/.

12. Michael Pollan, "Some of My Best Friends Are Germs," *New York Times,* May 15, 2013, https://www.nytimes.com/2013/05/19/magazine/say-hello-to-the-100-trillion-bacteria-that-make-up-your-microbiome.html.

6. CIRCADIAN FASTING

1. "The Nobel Prize in Physiology or Medicine 2017," NobelPrize.org, https://www.nobelprize.org/prizes/medicine/2017/summary/.

2. University of Basel, "Our Circadian Clock Sets the Rhythm for Our Cells' Powerhouses," ScienceDaily, March 6, 2018, https://www.sciencedaily.com/releases/2018/03/180306093116.htm.

3. Nicola Davis and Ian Sample, "Nobel Prize for Medicine Awarded for Insights into Internal Biological Clock," *Guardian,* October 2, 2017, https://www.theguardian.com/science/2017/oct/02/nobel-prize-for-medicine-awarded-for-insights-into-internal-biological-clock.

4. Rhonda Patrick, "Dr. Satchin Panda on Time-Restricted Feeding and Its Effects on Obesity, Muscle Mass and Heart Health," *FoundMyFitness* podcast, June 30, 2016, https://www.youtube.com/watch?v=-R-eqJDQ2nU.

5. AP, "Graveyard Shift Linked to Cancer Risk," NBCNews.com, November 29, 2007, http://www.nbcnews.com/id/22026660/ns/health-cancer/t/graveyard-shift-linked-cancer-risk/%23.VKrqXSfnLBc#.Xcq91ZJKjBo.

6. AP, "Graveyard Shift."

7. Katherine Brooks, "Is Blue Light the Bad Guy?" Right as Rain by UW Medicine, October 28, 2019, https://rightasrain.uwmedicine.org/well/health/blue-light.

8. Joshua J. Gooley et al., "Exposure to Room Light Before Bedtime Suppresses Melatonin Onset and Shortens Melatonin Duration in Humans," *Journal of Clinical Endocrinology and Metabolism* 96, no. 3 (March 2011): E463–E472, available at US National Library of Medicine, https://www.ncbi.nlm.nih.gov/pmc/articles/PMC3047226/.

9. Gabby Landsverk and Hilary Brueck, "Google Revealed the Top Trending Diet Searches of 2019, and It Included Plans from Celebrities like J. Lo and Adele," Insider, December 19, 2019, https://www.insider.com/most-popular-diets-2019-intermittent-fasting-noom-google-search-2019-12.

10. Michelle Harvie et al., "The Effect of Intermittent Energy and Carbohydrate Restriction v. Daily Energy Restriction on Weight Loss and Metabolic Disease Risk Markers in Overweight Women," *British Journal of Nutrition* 110, no. 8 (October 2013): 1534–47, available at US National Library of Medicine, https://www.ncbi.nlm.nih.gov/pubmed/23591120; Bronwen Martin et al., "Sex-Dependent Metabolic, Neuroendocrine, and Cognitive Responses to Dietary Energy Restriction and Excess," *Endocri-

nology 148, no. 9 (September 2007): 4318–33, available at US National Library of Medicine, https://www.ncbi.nlm.nih.gov/pubmed/17569758.

11. Rafael De Cabo and Mark P. Mattson, "Effects of Intermittent Fasting on Health, Aging, and Disease," *New England Journal of Medicine* 381, no. 26 (December 26, 2019): 2541–51, doi:10.1056/nejmra1905136.

12. De Cabo and Mattson, "Effects of Intermittent Fasting."

13. De Cabo and Mattson, "Effects of Intermittent Fasting."

14. De Cabo and Mattson, "Effects of Intermittent Fasting."

15. Catherine R. Marinac, Sandahl H. Nelson, Caitlin I. Breen, Sheri J. Hartman, Loki Natarajan, John P. Pierce, Shirley W. Flatt, Dorothy D. Sears, and Ruth E. Patterson, "Prolonged Nightly Fasting and Breast Cancer Prognosis," *JAMA Oncology* 2, no. 8 (August 1, 2016): 1049–55, available at US National Library of Medicine, https://www.ncbi.nlm.nih.gov/pmc/articles/PMC4982776/.

16. Bronwen Martin, Mark P. Mattson, and Stuart Maudsley, "Caloric Restriction and Intermittent Fasting: Two Potential Diets for Successful Brain Aging," *Ageing Research Reviews* 5, no. 3 (August 2006): 332–53, available at US National Library of Medicine, https://www.ncbi.nlm.nih.gov/pmc/articles/PMC2622429/.

17. Mo'ez Al-Islam E. Faris, Safia Kacimi, Ref'at A. Al-Kurd, Mohammad A. Fararjeh, Yasser K. Bustanji, Mohammad K. Mohammad, and Mohammad L. Salem, "Intermittent Fasting During Ramadan Attenuates Proinflammatory Cytokines and Immune Cells in Healthy Subjects," *Nutrition Research* 32, no. 12 (December 2012): 947–55, available at US National Library of Medicine, https://www.ncbi.nlm.nih.gov/pubmed/23244540.

18. De Cabo and Mattson, "Effects of Intermittent Fasting."

19. National Sleep Foundation, "How Age Affects Your Circadian Rhythm Changes," SleepFoundation.org, https://www.sleepfoundation.org/articles/how-age-affects-your-circadian-rhythm.

20. Sushil Kumar and Gurcharan Kuar, "Intermittent Fasting Dietary Restriction Regimen Negatively Influences Reproduction in Young Rats: A Study of Hypothalamo-Hypophysial-Gonadal Axis," *PloS One* 8, no. 1 (January 2013), available at US National Library of Medicine, https://www.ncbi.nlm.nih.gov/pubmed/23382817/.

21. Kumar and Kuar, "Intermittent Fasting Dietary Restriction Regimen."

7. ALL TOGETHER NOW

1. Michael J. Orlich et al., "Vegetarian Dietary Patterns and Mortality in Adventist Health Study 2," *JAMA Internal Medicine* 173, no. 13 (July 8, 2013): 1230–38, available at US National Library of Medicine, www.ncbi.nlm.nih.gov/pmc/articles/PMC4191896/.

2. Andrew Reynolds, Jim Mann, John Cummings, Nicola Winter, Evelyn Mete, and Lisa Te Morenga, "Carbohydrate Quality and Human Health: A Series of Systematic Reviews and Meta-Analyses," *Lancet* 393, no. 10170 (February 2, 2019): 434–45, available at US National Library of Medicine, https://www.ncbi.nlm.nih.gov/pubmed/30638909.

3. Meghan Jardine, "Seven Foods to Supercharge Your Gut Bacteria," Natural Health News, April 24, 2017, https://www.naturalhealthnews.uk/article/seven-foods-to-supercharge-your-gut-bacteria/.

4. Huadong Chen and Shengmin Sang, "Biotransformation of Tea Polyphenols by Gut Microbiota," *Journal of Functional Foods* 7 (March 2014): 26–42, available at ScienceDirect, https://www.sciencedirect.com/science/article/abs/pii/S1756464614000140.

5. Timothy Bond and Emma Derbyshire, "Tea Compounds and the Gut Microbiome: Findings from Trials and Mechanistic Studies," *Nutrients* 11, no. 10 (October 3, 2019): 2364, https://www.mdpi.com/2072-6643/11/10/2364/htm.

6. University College London, "Black Tea Soothes Away Stress," ScienceDaily, October 4, 2006, https://www.sciencedaily.com/releases/2006/10/061004173749.htm.

7. Joe Leech, "7 Science-Based Health Benefits of Drinking Enough Water," Healthline, June 4, 2017, https://www.healthline.com/nutrition/7-health-benefits-of-water#section2; Barry M. Popkin, Kristen E. D'Anci, and Irwin H. Rosenberg, "Water, Hydration, and Health," *Nutrition Reviews* 68, no. 8 (August 2010): 439–58, available at US National Library of Medicine, https://www.ncbi.nlm.nih.gov/pmc/articles/PMC2908954/.

8. "Alcohol and Arthritis," Arthritis Foundation, https://www.arthritis.org/living-with-arthritis/arthritis-diet/foods-to-avoid-limit/alcohol-in-moderation.php.

9. Jennifer Berry, "What Are the Health Benefits of Cardamom?," Medical News Today, October 2, 2019, https://www.medicalnewstoday.com/articles/326532.php.

10. M. Silvia Taga, E. E. Miller, and D. E. Pratt, "Chia Seeds as a Source of Natural Lipid Antioxidants," *Journal of the American Oil Chemists' Society* 61 (1984): 928–31, available at SpringerLink, link.springer.com/article/10.1007/BF02542169.

11. "Anti-Inflammatory Benefits of Flaxseed," *Living with Arthritis* (blog), May 4, 2016, Arthritis Foundation, http://blog.arthritis.org/living-with-arthritis/health-benefits-flaxseed-anti-inflammatory/.

12. "Turmeric and Dementia," Alzheimer's Society, https://www.alzheimers.org.uk/about-dementia/risk-factors-and-prevention/turmeric-and-dementia.

13. "Dirt Poor: Have Fruits and Vegetables Become Less Nutritious?" *Scientific American,* April 27, 2011, https://www.scientificamerican.com/article/soil-depletion-and-nutrition-loss/.

14. "How You Can Still Get Cancer (Even If You Live a Healthy Lifestyle)," The Hearty Soul, May 18, 2018, https://theheartysoul.com/pesticides-preservatives-raise-cancer-risk/.

15. H. Vally and N. L. Misso, "Adverse Reactions to the Sulphite Additives," *Gastroenterology and Hepatology from Bed to Bench* 5, no. 1 (2012): 16–23.

16. Consumer Reports, "Why You Don't Have to Give Up All Meat to Have a Healthy Diet," *Washington Post,* March 23, 2020, https://www.washingtonpost.com/health/why-you-dont-have-to-give-up-all-meat-to-have-a-healthy-diet/2020/03/20/bac262b2-5734-11ea-ab68-101ecfec2532_story.html.

17. Julieanna Hever, "Plant-Based Diets: A Physician's Guide," *Permanente Journal* 20, no. 3 (Summer 2016), https://www.thepermanentejournal.org/issues/2016/summer/6192-diet.html.

18. "Cancer Risk of Overcooked Meat Tested on Mice," NHS, November 4, 2011, https://www.nhs.uk/news/cancer/cancer-risk-of-overcooked-meat-tested-in-mice/.

19. Hever, "Plant-Based Diets."

20. Zeneng Wang et al., "Impact of Chronic Dietary Red Meat, White Meat, or Non-Meat Protein on Trimethylamine N-Oxide Metabolism and Renal Excretion in Healthy Men and Women," *European Heart Journal* 40, no. 7 (February 14, 2019): 583–94, available at Oxford Academic, academic.oup.com/eurheartj/article/40/7/583/5232723.

21. American Physiological Society, "Eat Your Vegetables (and Fish): Another Reason

Why They May Promote Heart Health," ScienceDaily, November 6, 2108, www.sci encedaily.com/releases/2018/11/181106073239.htm.

22. "Moderate Egg Intake Not Associated with Cardiovascular Disease Risk: Study," *British Medical Journal*, March 4, 2020, available at Medical Xpress, medicalxpress.com/news/2020-03-moderate-egg-intake-cardiovascular-disease.html.

23. "Fish: Friend or Foe?" Nutrition Source, Harvard School of Public Health, https://www.hsph.harvard.edu/nutritionsource/fish/.

24. Stacy Simon, "Soy and Cancer Risk: Our Expert's Advice," American Cancer Society, April 29, 2019, https://www.cancer.org/latest-news/soy-and-cancer-risk-our-experts -advice.html.

25. "Does Soy Boost Your Breast Cancer Risk?" Health Essentials, Cleveland Clinic, March 4, 2014, https://health.clevelandclinic.org/does-soy-boost-breast-cancer -risk/; Katherine Zeratsky, "Will Eating Soy Increase My Risk of Breast Cancer?" Healthy Lifestyle, Mayo Clinic, April 8, 2020, https://www.mayoclinic.org/healthy -lifestyle/nutrition-and-healthy-eating/expert-answers/soy-breast-cancer-risk/faq -20120377.

26. Heli E. K. Virtanen, Sari Voutilainen, Timo T. Koskinen, Jaakko Mursu, Tomi-Pekka Tuomainen, and Jyrki K. Virtanen, "Intake of Different Dietary Proteins and Risk of Heart Failure in Men," *Circulation: Heart Failure*, May 29, 2018, https://www.ahajour nals.org/doi/full/10.1161/circheartfailure.117.004531.

27. Virtanen et al., "Intake of Different Dietary Proteins."

28. Neda Seyedsadjadi, Jade Berg, Ayse A. Bilgin, Nady Braidy, Chris Salonikas, and Ross Grant, "High Protein Intake Is Associated with Low Plasma NAD+ Levels in a Healthy Human Cohort," *PloS One* 13, no. 8 (August 16, 2018), available at US National Library of Medicine, https://www.ncbi.nlm.nih.gov/pubmed/30114226.

29. "Shifts Needed to Align with Healthy Eating Patterns," chapter 2 of *Dietary Guidelines for Americans, 2015–2020*, 8th ed., https://health.gov/our-work/food-nutri tion/2015-2020-dietary-guidelines/guidelines/chapter-2/a-closer-look-at-current -intakes-and-recommended-shifts/.

30. Morgan E. Levine et al., "Low Protein Intake Is Associated with a Major Reduction in IGF-1, Cancer, and Overall Mortality in the 65 and Younger but Not Older Population," *Cell Metabolism* 19, no. 3 (March 4, 2014): 407–17, available at US National Library of Medicine, https://www.ncbi.nlm.nih.gov/pmc/articles/PMC3988204/.

8. GET WITH THE WTF PLAN

1. Alessa Nas, Nora Mirza, Franziska Hägele, Julia Kahlhöfer, Judith Keller, Russell Rising, Thomas A. Kufer, and Anja Bosy-Westphal, "Impact of Breakfast Skipping Compared with Dinner Skipping on Regulation of Energy Balance and Metabolic Risk," *American Journal of Clinical Nutrition* 105, no. 6 (June 2017): 1351–61, Oxford Academic, https://academic.oup.com/ajcn/article/105/6/1351/4668664.

2. "The Facts on Intermittent Fasting," Ms.Medicine, August 15, 2019, https://msmedi cine.com/the-facts-on-intermittent-fasting/.

3. Arnold Kahn and Anders Olsen, "Stress to the Rescue: Is Hormesis a 'Cure' for Aging?" *Dose-Response* 8, no. 1 (2010): 48–52, available at US National Library of Medicine, https://www.ncbi.nlm.nih.gov/pmc/articles/PMC2836152/.

4. Mark Sisson, "Hormesis: How Certain Kinds of Stress Can Actually Be Good for You," Mark's Daily Apple, https://www.marksdailyapple.com/hormesis-how-certain -kinds-of-stress-can-actually-be-good-for-you/.

5. Kate E. Lee, Kathryn J. H. Williams, Leisa D. Sargent, Nicholas S. G. Williams, and Katherine A. Johnson, "40-Second Green Roof Views Sustain Attention: The Role of Micro-Breaks in Attention Restoration," *Journal of Environmental Psychology* 42 (June 2015): 182–89, available at ScienceDirect, https://www.sciencedirect.com/science/article/abs/pii/S0272494415000328.

6. Patrick Ewers, "Want a Happier, More Fulfilling Life? 75-Year Harvard Study Says Focus on This 1 Thing," Pocket, https://getpocket.com/explore/item/want-a-happier-more-fulfilling-life-75-year-harvard-study-says-focus-on-this-1-thing?utm_source=pocket-newtab.

7. "Yoga Could Slow the Harmful Effects of Stress and Inflammation," *Harvard Health Blog*, October 19, 2017, www.health.harvard.edu/blog/yoga-could-slow-the-harmful-effects-of-stress-and-inflammation-2017101912588.

8. K. Uvnäs-Moberg, L. Handlin, and M. Petersson, "Self-Soothing Behaviors with Particular Reference to Oxytocin Release Induced by Non-Noxious Sensory Stimulation," *Frontiers in Psychology* 5 (2015): 1529, https://doi.org/10.3389/fpsyg.2014.01529.

10. ENER-CHI

1. University of Pittsburgh Schools of the Health Sciences, "New Insights into How the Mind Influences the Body," ScienceDaily, August 15, 2016, https://www.sciencedaily.com/releases/2016/08/160815185555.htm.

2. "The Brain-Gut Connection," Johns Hopkins Medicine, https://www.hopkinsmedicine.org/health/wellness-and-prevention/the-brain-gut-connection.

3. Eric Johnson, "Self-Help Author Tim Ferriss Says Social Media Is Making Us Miserable," Vox, January 23, 2017, https://www.vox.com/2017/1/23/14353880/tim-ferriss-tools-of-titans-4-hour-workweek-social-media-recode-podcast; "One Tech Investor on Why You Should Take a Break from Social Media," *Here & Now*, WBUR, February 8, 2017, https://www.wbur.org/hereandnow/2017/02/08/tim-ferriss.

4. Ben Bryant, "Judges Are More Lenient After Taking a Break, Study Finds," *Guardian*, April 11, 2011, https://www.theguardian.com/law/2011/apr/11/judges-lenient-break.

5. Eva M. Krockow, "How Many Decisions Do We Make Each Day?" *Psychology Today*, September 27, 2018, https://www.psychologytoday.com/us/blog/stretching-theory/201809/how-many-decisions-do-we-make-each-day#.

6. Jamison Monroe, "Understanding the Mind-Body Connection," Newport Academy, October 7, 2019, https://www.newportacademy.com/resources/mental-health/understanding-the-mind-body-connection/.

7. University of Plymouth, "Weight Loss Can Be Boosted Fivefold Thanks to Novel Mental Imagery Technique," ScienceDaily, September 24, 2018, https://www.sciencedaily.com/releases/2018/09/180924095729.htm.

8. "FoundMyFitness Topic — Sauna," FoundMyFitness, www.foundmyfitness.com/topics/sauna.

9. "Kuopio Ischaemic Heart Disease Risk Factor Study (KIHD, 1984–)," University of Eastern Finland, https://www.uef.fi/en/web/nutritionepidemiologists/kuopio-ischaemic-heart-disease-risk-factor-study-kihd-1984-.

10. Setor K. Kunutsor, Hassan Khan, Tanjaniina Laukkanen, and Jari A. Laukkanen, "Joint Associations of Sauna Bathing and Cardiorespiratory Fitness on Cardiovascular and All-Cause Mortality Risk: A Long-Term Prospective Cohort Study," *Annals of*

Medicine 50, no. 2 (March 2018): 139–46, available at US National Library of Medicine, https://www.ncbi.nlm.nih.gov/pubmed/28972808.

11. JAMA Network Journals, "Sauna Use Associated with Reduced Risk of Cardiac, All-Cause Mortality," February 23, 2015, ScienceDaily, www.sciencedaily.com/releases/2015/02/150223122602.htm.

12. Tanjaniina Laukkanen, Setor K. Kunutsor, Hassan Khan, Peter Willeit, Francesco Zaccardi, and Jari A. Laukkanen, "Sauna Bathing Is Associated with Reduced Cardiovascular Mortality and Improves Risk Prediction in Men and Women: A Prospective Cohort Study," *BMC Medicine* 16 (2018): 219, available at US National Library of Medicine, https://www.ncbi.nlm.nih.gov/pmc/articles/PMC6262976/.

13. Lisa Rapaport, "Regular Sauna Users May Have Fewer Chronic Diseases," Reuters, August 1, 2018, https://www.reuters.com/article/us-health-sauna/regular-sauna-users-may-have-fewer-chronic-diseases-idUSKBN1KM5U0.

14. Carole A. Baggerly et al., "Sunlight and Vitamin D: Necessary for Public Health," *Journal of the American College of Nutrition* 34, no. 4 (July 4, 2015): 359–65, available at US National Library of Medicine, https://www.ncbi.nlm.nih.gov/pmc/articles/PMC4536937/.

15. Megan Buerger, "Stressed Out? Here Are 10 Science-Backed Design Tips for Bringing Serenity to Your Home," *Washington Post*, August 28, 2019, https://www.washingtonpost.com/lifestyle/home/stressed-out-here-are-10-science-backed-design-tips-for-bringing-serenity-to-your-home/2019/08/27/187e362e-c50e-11e9-b72f-b31dfaa77212_story.html.

16. Ingrid Fetell Lee, "7 Ways to Reduce Anxiety in Your Home Through Design," The Aesthetics of Joy, https://aestheticsofjoy.com/2016/11/02/5747/.

17. Darby Saxbe and Rena L. Repetti, "For Better or Worse? Coregulation of Couples' Cortisol Levels and Mood States," *Journal of Personality and Social Psychology* 98, no. 1 (January 2010): 92–103, available at US National Library of Medicine, https://www.ncbi.nlm.nih.gov/pubmed/20053034.

18. Admiral William H. McRaven (Ret.), *Make Your Bed: Little Things That Can Change Your Life . . . and Maybe the World* (New York: Grand Central, 2017).

19. Shubhra Krishan, *Essential Ayurveda: What It Is and What It Can Do for You* (Novato, CA: New World Library, 2003), 3.

Further Reading

As I mentioned in the book, there is no shortage of information about hormones, and the information seems to grow daily. If you want to dig deeper on our hormonal system, here are a few books I recommend for further reading:

Will Bulsiewicz, MD, *Fiber Fueled: The Plant-Based Gut Health Program for Losing Weight, Restoring Your Health, and Optimizing Your Microbiome*

Jason Fung, MD, *The Obesity Code: Unlocking the Secrets of Weight Loss*

Sara Gottfried, MD, *The Hormone Cure: Reclaim Balance, Sleep, and Sex Drive; Lose Weight; Feel Focused, Vital, and Energized Naturally with the Gottfried Protocol*

John R. Lee, MD, *Dr. John Lee's Hormone Balance Made Simple: The Essential How-to Guide to Symptoms, Dosage, Timing, and More*

Christiane Northrup, MD, *The Wisdom of Menopause: Creating Physical and Emotional Health During the Change*

Aviva Romm, MD, *The Adrenal Thyroid Revolution: A Proven 4-Week Program to Rescue Your Metabolism, Hormones, Mind and Mood*

Index

Page numbers in *italics* refer to illustrations.

hydration, 145, 156, 188
hydrogenated oils, 164
hypercortisolism, 39–42
hyperinsulinemia, 178
hyperpigmentation, 42–43
hyperthermia, 289
hyperthyroidism, 30, 32–33
hypocortisolism, 42–43
hypothalamic-pituitary-adrenal
    axis (HPA), 22, 24, 119
hypothalamus, 11, 26–28, 30,
    122
hypothyroidism, 30–32

immune system, 11, 15, 105–7,
    110–11, 179–80
indole-3-carbinol, 67
inflammation
    acute, 80
    brain and, 85
    causes of, 84
    chronic, 80–81
    correcting, 89–101
    diet and, 12, 85–86, 89–98
    energy trifecta and, 81–83
    fatigue and, 85–86
    fish and, 169
    foods good for, 175
    function of, 79–80
    immune system and, 11
    leaky gut and, 88–89
    omega-3s and, 160
    omega-6s and, 165
    plant-based diets and,
        151–52
    signs of, 83–85
    superfoods and, 157–59
    tea and, 154–55
    weight gain and, 86–88
    yoga and, 212
inflammatory bowel disease
    (IBD), 155
inner calm, 190–91
insoluble fiber, 150
insulin, 25, 26, 33–34, 62, 165,
    180
insulin resistance, 34–36, 87,
    173, 180
insulin-like growth hormone
    factor 1 (IGF-1), 131,
    168, 174
intermittent fasting (IF). See
    circadian/intermittent
    fasting
International Agency for
    Research on Cancer
    (IARC), 164
interval training, 100
intestinal permeability, 109. See
    also leaky gut
iodine, 29
isoflavones, 167, 170

Journal of Environmental
    Psychology, 206

Kale-Chard Salad with Creamy
    Cashew Dressing,
    233–34
Kebabs, Moong Dal, 268

mucin, 91, 116
Muffins, Banana Oatmeal, 227
myenteric plexus, 110

Naan, Gluten-Free, 273–74
Nachos, Healthy, 246–47
NAD levels, 174
napping, 145
National Institute of Environ-
     mental Health Sciences,
     82
nature, 99–100, 206–7, 290
negative chronic inflammation,
     11
negative thoughts, 284–85
negative/toxic people, 283–84
neurotransmitters, 107–8
neurotrophic growth factor,
     128
New England Journal of Medicine,
     129, 130–31, 149
N-glycolylneuraminic acid
     (Neu5Gc), 168
night shifts, 124–25
nitrates, 164
noradrenaline, 37
norepinephrine, 37
NSAIDs, 114
nut milks, 167

oats
     Banana Oatmeal Muffins,
          227
     Cocoa-Oat Prebiotic Break-
          fast Bars, 228

Vegetable-Oats Dosa,
     269–70
oils, 165–66
Okra Masala, 265–66
omega-3s, 19, 95, 158, 160, 163,
     165, 169, 172
omega-6s, 165–66, 172
One Meal a Day (OMAD),
     135
One-Pan Roasted Asparagus
     and Brussels Sprouts,
     248–49
Orange-Cardamom Chia Seed
     Pudding, 225
organic foods, 62
ovaries, 23
oxidative stress, 92
oxytocin, 27

pancreas, 23, 64
pancreatic hormones, 33–36
Panda, Satchin, 64, 136
pantry staples, 218–19, 221
parabens, 65, 66, 67–68, 101,
     210
parasympathetic nervous sys-
     tem, 72, 76–77
Parfaits, Cannoli, 277–78
pasteurization, 93, 166
Penne "Alfredo" with Roasted
     Cauliflower, 256–57
pepper, 159–60
peptic ulcer disease (PUD),
     155
perimenopause, 44, 47, 65–66

About the Author

Amy Shah, MD, is a double-board-certified medical doctor and wellness expert specializing in allergy/immunology, hormones, and gut health. Dr. Shah graduated magna cum laude from Cornell University's School of Nutrition and went on to receive her medical doctorate with distinction in research at Albert Einstein Medical College. She completed her residency and fellowship at the Harvard and Columbia hospital systems. She lives in Paradise Valley, Arizona, with her husband and two children. This is her first book.